CORRUPTION OF VIROLOGY INSTIGATES DEHUMANIZATION

DR. WISDOM C. GWATIDZO

authorHOUSE®

AuthorHouse™
1663 Liberty Drive
Bloomington, IN 47403
www.authorhouse.com
Phone: 833-262-8899

Published by AuthorHouse 11/03/2020

ISBN: 978-1-6655-0612-0 (sc)
ISBN: 978-1-6655-0610-6 (hc)
ISBN: 978-1-6655-0611-3 (e)

Library of Congress Control Number: 2020921349

Print information available on the last page.

All scriptures were taken from the King James version of the Bible.

CONTENTS

DEDICATIONS

I dedicate this walked-upon story to my only begotten son God gave upon my loins, affectionately Jemu, from the Book of James, whose tears (as he suffered with me) many found hard to stop, as they required the key/tap to be stirred upon the source - the heart! And of a TRUTH, The LORD could have well-meant my travail for a father & son's closer walk with Him on the narrow way to 'Moriah' for that perfect sacrifice of substitution - The Lamb of Redemption. Future conversations should be listened to one another from the ear in the bosom.

I also dedicate it to God's love in the Mother of the womb and breasts and hands that fed me. Not forgetting the amazing sons God gave directly from the link heaven.com, even my beloved

Frank, and his younger brothers God gave to learn and follow, even Tino the loyal & obedient time-keeper (Tinotenda) and our 'New' the blessed nourisher (Newton). And the rest of our executive team members, Anè the wonderful cross-checker(Anesu), Inno my young-brother & friend (Innocent) and Tiri the prayed-for-nephew (Zephaniah). How can I forget the well-meant doctors, beloved Issy (Israel), and the gifted Chris (Christopher), both never to be swayed from a dedicated & earnest practice.

Last but not least, I dedicate his book, to our never-grow-old Gogo in the garden (Gogo Mazanhanga). Then again to rope around all these dedications, I draw upon the Lord's belt of Love in the fore-gone parents of practical charity and answered-prayer preserved in God's Golden Vessel, even Rev Titus E. Shamba and Woman-Pastor Mrs E. Zvanyanya; and prayerful partakers still remaining with us to this day,even Mukoma (Rev E Mutsambwa-Moyo) and Atate the humble Preaching Prayer Warrior (Baba Luckson Amon Banda).

AUTHOR'S PREFACE

The world is changing. It has ever been doing so. But presently it is changing fast and even drastically at times. As the world is changing, it is helpful to be aware of the central reason for change: Is it due to the Supreme-being? Or it is due to the human-being? In one of his statements, the remarkable preacher – John Wesley of renown warned: 'Do not hastily attribute everything to God!'

Some years back, while on a field trip, our team happened to pass through a naturally-fenced horticulture garden of a villager – whose works demonstrated – he was an intelligent and diligent worker beyond adequate description! He had a practical map of his garden in relation to soil and especially wetness of areas. In his brief introduction, he highlighted, how each zone had transformed to bear less water over decades, leading to 'dead' previous marshes and birth of previously non-existing dry areas – therefore all areas now demanded irrigation! I asked him why they suffered such a change and he answered with no jot of delay: '**The world is changing.**' His confident frank face already indicated he was not going to add more words – it was enough – we all heard it – and we all swallowed quietly!

I reflected as we trudged on. The term '**climate change**' had not yet so prominently dawned, though it was most probably 'around the corner'. Soon we were to learn of the hazards of climate change in comments in almost every workshop by mention of risk factors if not the actual theme.

But such a change, though the impact was to weigh with seeming sudden heaviness, crept on much slower.

COVID (rightly attached a numerical suffix 19 by way of agreement if not disagreement of times) has not been like that – indeed it has been like drastic, a change in the turn of a decade and the century bearing it!

Sad to say, that like climate change, a phenomena which could possibly have been thought to be of Nature, it is also quite unnatural, and deadly artificial, pointing to the adulterous wedlock of western and eastern blocks' laboratory sciences – the proven 'new-age' deadly virology of times and its threatening tail and trail of vaccination!

A question came to me, not even as an author, but even before I ever thought to write: Who is meant to be eliminated by who out of the balance of Access to Benefit Sharing? Who is superior beyond the plan of the Creator to think beyond Divine intelligence? Where is this human planner of super-guided 'pandemics' who is probably dangerously trying to mimic Moses' God-granted powers to bring plagues during the era of the hardened Pharaoh? And he is happy to confuse the apparent 'Christian-world' to pray and sing that the end-times are near if not here?

Yes the end times are near, but the sin of mimicry by men, shall find its owner, be careful, possibly even before the end comes!

Now, the reality of COVID, is there, and in the corruption of the ages, as perpetrated through viruses and vaccinations, is ravaging massacres in the West, North and East! Africa has not been spared of the corruption, and in its ripe and ready corrupt environment, it is the platform of this real literature, to demonstrate how she has flared and fared in this short era – before the real COVID's entrance into many of her unjustified and unfortunate subdivisions of nations!

To my brethren of Africa, and its busy-bodies of 'frontline-panners', I have warned: 'WATCH OUT – THE REAL COVID IS COMING!' And by the way, when it's fully come, no 'gold panner' will wait on its way, permitting only the true front-liner worker – the dedicated caregiver, never money-driven – but fuelled ever by the love and care for humanity! How many are left in Africa? Or how many have not left their Africa?

Read and follow slowly, and the whole meaning shall be revealed to you – my dear Reader!

FOREWORD

(Sins have tails of trails like the disdainful snail-trail)

1 Timothy 5v24 says: 'Some men's sins are open beforehand, going before to judgment; and **some men they follow after.**'

The sins of those men who planned the HIV era of corruption in Virology and ugly-Vaccination, again originating in the laboratory, and now evidently almost officially convicted, of their cruel destruction and murder of African generations, effecting 'orphaning' and 'widowing', to a cycle of further destruction of these inevitable remnants unto innumerable ruins void of living laughter amid villages - such sins indeed left a trail seemingly to be forever hidden then as in an ocean, but to be revealed like a mountain today!

These same virulent sinners of virology, at the time, with much deceit and cover-ups, thought they would be in a lifetime's 'hideout'. They did not realize in time that as they would endeavor to kill more, a tail would be growing to reveal them more, bearing sacs of poison in the disguise of vaccines as the COVID era upset their engineering of genes beyond the human and fetal tissue menace, revealing even their past sins with vivid openness! COVID even seems bound to be threatening to present more tentacles and horns in the way of sin-protrusions, before they themselves polish to disguise the rotten insides of their destructive marketing of child-adult menacing inoculations! Will the dullest among the African populations be fooled – let brethren help brethren into light!

Now, no one loves to see snails in their garden! Unfortunately, certain from the Eastern world, during their migrations in Africa, have ended up breeding them for strange appetites, leading to townships teeming with clusters of them like balls and boulders within the gardens and yards of the locals – an unpleasant situation indeed. The slimy trails of snails in the COVID corruption, track all the way from the Western and Eastern blocks of Science and Economics, all the way down to Africa of simplicity, even with links such as the WHO in between! Corruption in the home, in the workplace, in the worship place, and even now in the lockdown-proven useless entertainment centre, is disgusting! But if someone designs/engineers a corrupted virus and a matching corrupt vaccine, to wipe away populations in a corrupting cycle that spins worldwide to eliminate with segregation, that trail of sin by such a person has currently been proven in the Wisdom of the Creator to even turn against his own, and his own shall judge him first, before the helpless have been wiped – and the Scripture seals it for time: '...your sin will find you out'.

The pattern in the first world and China, demonstrates ignorance in the seeming most learned professors, from being deceived into unrealistic patterns of false pathophysiology defined as a range from flu/cough – up to Respiratory Distress Syndrome (RDS), till real observations of blood-clots, emboli, mucus obstructions, allergic reactions, hyper-inflammation, bleeding disorders with hypoxia of not such a type to be aided by 'common' use of ventilators but to be worsened by it! And reality of more observations still flows in, with discolorations of extremities as though measles lesions. Amid this confusion, death is raging and reigning so badly that the frontline staff tremble to this day.

Meanwhile in Africa, the situation is still quite different to this day of writing (17th of May 2020), with most cases being incidental findings of positive tests, based on nasopharyngeal swabs for PCR, never calibrated for the African population but for the Eastern bloc where the seeming donation in kind came from – and with interesting stories of false positives in sheep and goats and even most laughably on a watermelon to bring a lot of doubt of authenticity in the minds of true scientists. Now how many are true scientists in Africa? Or there are mostly certificate holders who are ready unthinking slaves for the pharmaceutical kingdom with their pens to make prescriptions of any drug or vaccine or substance that the 'master' claims!

This early hour, the corruption trail is on a different note somehow! Some 'hawks' among the frontline workers have realized how to capture 'checks' (not chicks this time around) without the threat of the contagion of COVID. They spot the false positive cases, which are obviously non-threatening and currently the majority – establish as many contacts as possible for follow-up of these sure-to turnout-negative cases, and earn as much money before real COVID of described killing features above, dawns! And they trouble sufferers, really ill of Malaria, Cancer, Pneumonia or other serious afflictions, whilst painstakingly visiting without fail and claiming even the so-called T & S from overtime and late-night visits from the contacts very much unlikely or never to suffer from COVID! And it is to these 'gold panners', to whom I have said: 'LET REAL COVID COME – AND NON OF YOU COWARDS IN CORRUPTION SHALL REMAIN IN THE FRONTLINE, BY WAY OF DEATH OR TEMPORARY HIDING! And so it is, the delay in the real dawn of the real COVID, has promoted such corruption to this day in the Southern part of the African Continent! Yet the virology-fathers and vaccine-owners of this corruption-trail, residing in the North and Western zone, with allies in the daily-corrupt East, are ignorant of this pre-COVID brew full of yeast and various catalysts to spin and move their alternative of busy-body counterparts down of the Equator – and both parties one day shall pay the price of one's own part!

Let us get into the active story now, dear Reader, lest you be tempted to sleep – wake up, it's not yet time to slumber!

CHAPTER ONE

—— ✿ ——

INTRODUCTION

Corruption akin to the deadly virus

There is a naturally existing virus from Creation. But there are corrupt Scientists, from the body called virologists, who can now corrupt that naturally existing virus, into a harmful and lethal one, for an evil motive, intent or purpose on a segregated population, whether tribe, nation, race or creed! Such a purpose is usually to kill and not just to maim – to decimate populations – who doesn't know such agenda, unless he deliberately doesn't want to know?!

And at the top, the laboratory level, the sins are first class; and though they involve a few, yet that's the beginning of the tap-root. All the accessory roots spreading around the corruption-tree's world are second to third class and even lower. Hence at the Centre of the intention to kill, there will be great sinners of a huge coverage in their accomplishment as an aeroplane. Meanwhile at the villages/communities to be slaughtered, there too exists an exercise and will to kill by kinsmen, trained along the strategy of the first-class sinners. The latter, soon or later, get to know that their job may kill, but they are covered and showered with the evil cover-up blessing of money – the root of all evil. So you hear such lower accessory & support root-level workers: 'Guys, let's go out for money, this is our opportunity, our golden chance, it may never come again!' Indeed they mean it, and they stiffen their backs to the thought of what they truly know.

I would like to dwell on these latter lower-level frontline executors if not executioners, their zeal, their lack of real fear but possessed by a fictitious flare for fear, their lack of expertise in the invasiveness of procedures - especially the nasopharyngeal swab, their lack of care, and lastly the fact that they will do nothing for you to earn life – even a bottle of good water! They even add burdens onto those patients already suffering from other ailments/afflictions and not long to label them COVID soonest as the test returns – upon which they start treating them like sacks of sand or logs. Kindness, love, compassion, mercy, long-suffering and patience are taboo to their hearts.

They are all woven, knitted and linked in behavior in that network from the hospitals down to the villages. Those at the hospital boot out in derision and scorn, whilst those visiting the villages kick at and laugh at. The latter are very interesting, they hardly miss a visit in this money-driven scheme, if not scandal of lockdowns. We shall dwell more upon this later on. All in all, if these latter lower earners do something great for you – it is the taking of a temperature, and currently they are excited if not exhilarated by the infrared-gunner – which they point as though they are proudly equipped to shoot – thank God at least they can read the numbers that come out on the screen. The rest, after taking of the temperatures is to try to engage you in chatting. One of them bolted out a smartphone in an attempt to shoot out videos – I immediately and effectively reprimanded him and stopped him.

At this point, let me briefly bring you to the medical team, usually of two doctors who come especially to prod the swab into your nasopharyngeal passage and twist a number of times without guided strength upon the mucosal lining that links with the para-nasal air-sinuses – injury or inflammation, as of immediate or long-term complications, who cares!?!? We shall talk more of that too!

Then they make a schedule; and even if one may understand that anyone may fail to abide by it, but at least any professional should apologize in time, and propose another day and time, trying to ensure it won't fail. Then this postponement gets onto auto-drive, without care that a person, supposed to be in self-quarantine for 21 days, to be freed by a negative swab/PCR test, is now beyond a week in excess of the due-date – he suffers it all with risk of stress and physical and psychosocial exacerbation as he is afraid to be labelled a fugitive by the 'security-doctors', and might compromise his 'freedom' or the quality thereof from such 'superiors' at the end of it all – that is if it ever comes to a real end. Enjoyment of power, one just doesn't understand?! Or may be seeking a bribe to spice upon the kills of the season, who knows?! But all the same, this is the game, and match-fixing could be more comprehensible.

Then, the security of your life is in their hands. They have invasive access to your special areas so much in proximity with channels to your brain – and should any one of them, security doctors, decide on his behalf or someone else's, to introduce an inoculum or a slow-killing substance into your cavities, you are weak to oppose – forces may be taken to subdue you – and you are defenseless! In most cases, there is hardly any room for an assay at a private lab, the program having been the 'rightful' download on the global 'viro-lineage', from the north down south.

Then what if someone decides to make your result positive on paper – what will you do – results being ushered via a special security channel too? Will it help to protest? Better would it be, if a private lab out of the sphere of the program's influence would avail cross-checking. And how many will afford on the village class to pay for themselves, let alone just to shout, but may be to sob or weep! And at the end of the day, mothers crying for their sons have no one to hear them, sons crying for their own fathers seem silent in a lockdown world, daughters without protection are possibly the most vulnerable, while grandparents, previously supported, cry for their supporter. But then this is Africa and no one has a fund at hand to hand over to them; if at all some money or donations had flown for the program - it has gotten into the pockets of the smart – another virus – 'COVID (II)'!

Now the social media – some official, medical very possible, may have an omission of ethics in the excitement, start a chat with a non-medical friend – the result can be a 'forest-fire'! In one of our native languages – Shona – who doesn't know our gift of a proverb: '*Kamoto kamberevere kanopisa matanda mberi*', which is literally, '**a small flame can be the herald of a veld-fire's devastation of a logging harvest**'. In the end, there will even be false death reports by social-media participants at the vegetable market, in possession of smartphones: 'that so-and-so has died from COVID' – a painful experience for some limelight figures who may suffer image-tarnishing even to the affection of their jobs and movements. Yet all this corruption has a head, and don't forget, if the tail is not yet seen, it shall appear. The epicenter of the vibrations may be there up in the North and West and East, but the tremors are not missed down in the southerly villages. So is the case with COVID 19 and the corruption strands about it!

CHAPTER TWO

———— ✎ ————

ADMISSION

The incidental finding of a 'positive' test reigns

The signs and science around my illness objectively

I was admitted at the Central Hospital on the 24th of April 2020. It was a Friday night. The morning had seen a check Malaria test positive, initially the parasitaemia assayed to be 2.8% (previous result one week back was 2.7%). The test on this day had been meant to check if I had improved on a very special therapy from our NFH service for about a week's period, having started an even more special aspect of the therapy on April 2020 (details of which shall follow later on). On both occasions I had drawn blood on my own, first time into an EDTA tube, without any hassle or hardship or glimpse of failure – here I'm not hinting at my adeptness, but rather the following fact: I was still sound and my blood volume allowed me to do it on my own so easily.

It is vital that I conclude about the tests for Malaria at this point in time, in order to put things together. The consultant doctor at the laboratory of renown, did something extra-remarkable on the day. He phoned me sometime in the end of the day, I remember his compassionate kind voice:

'Dr Gwatidzo, is that Dr Gwatidzo Wisdom I'm speaking to – I need to speak to Dr Gwatidzo?', and after my affirmation he proceeded.

'Dr Gwatidzo, I have taken your blood sample and reanalyzed it myself, and realized that your parasitaemia has actually reached 20% instead, and I've done a Full Blood Count (FBC), demonstrating your haemoglobin (Hb) to be 13.5, not so bad though, but the platelets are scaringly down to 53!'

I thanked and informed him well, that I was on my way to be admitted, and my two colleagues, whom I had trained with, one I nickname Best-of-Surgeons (short cut BOS'), and the other now a specialist physician of great renown, were preparing to receive me for admission to start special treatment. He received my message and special thanksgiving with comfort and rest of mind. He wasn't far from sending these results to these friends of mine, the two doctors. By the way, he had done the extra-check at his own initiative and at the lab's own cost. Whether someone, a worker in their lab had hinted to him of my predicament from the tests, that: *'One of our service-providers who sends us patient-specimens consistently over the years* (now in my 28th year of practice) *seemeth very unwell from Malaria'*, that much I wouldn't know, but this lab head's practical compassion, I would remind The Lord to remember forever!

One thing that the lab doctor's references would never tell him, was my oxygen carrying capacity when I'm normal. For instance, my usual haemoglobin level is usually around 17 (+/- 1). This would mean in actual fact that about a third of this oxygen carrying capacity had been lost from my system, and indeed, post admission, the signs showed as I shall reveal later on. The platelets, so falling low, could lead to complications, including a tendency to bleed and other sinister complex complications on top of complications. Thank God, I was in good hands, and there was going to be no delay.

Cascade of events on the day of admission

Sorry dear reader, for pouring in too much of figures and parameters above, I wish it wasn't so much of a boring passage to pass in your reading. Anyway, let's get to an exciting cruise for now:

The morning on the admission day, had tale-tell signs whilst still at home in our richly naturally oxygenated Garden Centre, 88km out of the Capital City, amidst the villages and mountains. I had by now, been sleeping amidst two kindest of lads, each one of us on his own couch, and

I in the middle one; they were my helpers and guards (not from enemies) lest I fall, upon my initial effort to walk especially, after alighting to go to relieve via pressured sphincters. I shall indeed relate interesting episodes that remind me of very much telling proverbs in the vernacular!

Upon waking up that morning, we breakfasted upon our Bible reading as usual, and God blessed us with a wonderful prayer session overall – unknowing that the day would end with my temporary separation from my dear compassionate young friends. I'm 52 and they are both 23 now, in this famous year of 2020.

After prayer, things were moving very fast – I opted to go to the Corner House, a special guest house of memories in our Garden Centre, where God visits us often with unforgettable signs and wonders. Fortunately I had no pain anywhere in my body (I shall show how God dealt with the serious headache way-back, from the falciparum malaria's cerebral inflammation and irritation).

My greatest challenge had shown itself clearly by then: an extremely dry tongue which could surprisingly with the help of the vocal chords and bellows (lungs) still complain: '*I don't understand why I'm not producing any saliva!*' indeed not salivating, and this had been going on for maybe a week now, and had no idea how any pathophysiology of the medical realm would explain it. Urine I was passing, and frequently with reasonable color(s), as a 'new lover' of ice-cold water – strange, and so scarcely could I guess that I could be grossly dehydrated.

So up I went to the Corner house, steadily and very comfortably, alone, without support of my friends, entered in and gently got tucked under the warmth of linen in this well-ventilated room of super-comfort. I lavished the warmth and the serenity, and little did I realize that I was losing consciousness as the sun appeared to cruise faster than all the other days, as I took and felt everything for sleep in solace, only waking up here and there to throw urine.

A phone call came, and it was my beloved nephew, to confirm the results of that unimproved parasitaemia on the sample that I had drawn in the presence of my most-beloved son, Frank, that morning, who had in turn driven halfway before the capital city, to hand it to my nephew to take to the lab in the capital in the company of one of our dedicated workers. I agreed, on the phone, that it was time to go to the hospital, furthermore, it appeared now I couldn't eat or even drink much – a state which I slid into like the moon into the western horizon on a cold night.

Yet, by this hour of announcement of results, I was creeping lower in consciousness and interest in precise time, sinking gently into sweet deeper sleep each moment of passing daytime. Then suddenly there was an arrival, of familiar sweet voices, as 'the rescue team' of our own 'soldiers' had come – I only saw the brilliance as of the afternoon sun, yet hours had gone.

And I felt the 'hip-hip', 'let's go guys', and the lifting upon my matress seemingly so much easy for them, to be carried to our 'small-car' (thank God for its return from our great and faithful mechanic), about 50metres down the way. I felt most comfortable, above the hands of those that loved me. Something very significantly of interest: Over this 50metre stretch, I must have waken about 15 times, but falling again immediately into deep sleep, yet with comfort – then I felt the arrival by that rear car door of the nearside – and in they slid me as though I was on a lubricated slider – seemed so much easy for them – yah sure – Proverbs 20v29 tells it all…..
'The glory of young men is their strength….'

Immediately as the couch received me well, I felt something, of that particular sphincter every adult is very careful the most about – and I signaled: *'Ndinoda kwa Mukoma Frank'*, meaning I needed relief in the special ever-welcoming restroom in Bro Frank's lovely 'allowable' guesthouse. Innocent would not allow me to trudge and 'giddy' alone up the way, neither would Frank either, and I didn't take any notice of their close walk behind me until the glass-door. There I insisted: 'Oh no please, I can make it alone', yet after finishing the special discharge, I saw them waiting for me right inside Mukoma Frank's room as I opened the closet's door to leave. I felt much better, with great relief demonstrable even by my steady strides towards the small car – got myself into the car and lay myself down, covered myself with my warm jacket and automatically was deep. I think the ignition I heard, but the 400metres down to the tarmac was like a dream. And I remember the entry upon the tarmac – and indeed the journey had seriously begun. 'Hu-uu-uu-uu-uu, gunduru-gunduru-gunduru', I would hear the rhyming and echoing sounds as the small car cruised – I think Zeph's foot had the best footwear for a grip upon the *a*-paddle for the moment! Here and there, I would wake up, and see trees; surprisingly it was already dusk, in front of the light-greyish background of a welcome night, waving to me and sending me to 'sleep again'. I particularly remember three wakes, one about the 10km peg away from home, climbing up the uphill from the history-making bridge of Chivake river, and the 'bye-bying' trees did their job perfectly. I then woke up again at the halfway 'town' – not so comfortable with an impatient policeman at that 'lockdown' roadblock; by the way, the police officer at the 'lockdown' block just after home, had been very compassionate and just allowed us to 'slice' through, having been told it was I, and that the young men were rushing me to my awaiting colleagues at the 'big' hospital. The third remarkable awake, which saw me with most awake episodes up to the destination, was the negotiation of the roundabout past the shining Chisipite shopping mall – and the lights of the city seemed to hammer-in, the wake-up call – I think my mind condescended this time, and closed eyes no more meant sleep any longer. I even assisted to some extent on the familiar drive-route, all the way to the hospital – stolen a little bit before the hospital-gate entry point – overheard the guys discussing about which entrance to use, and I saw them take the correct one and acknowledged. Down and straight to the corner we went, as I heard them confirm arrival to my medical friend (even this bridegroom's wedding friend to witness on the marriage certificate). And Israel in his kind voice ever, affirmed he would soon be there. Faithful to his word as usual, he was just in time – went inside to see and organize the best way through the procedural initial stages of admission.

Here we go out from the car now

Just like one arriving in a new city, may get a little thought-ache: 'how shall I get there, am I sure of the directions I was given, will I be able to follow them, wish someone would assist me......?I'

So it was with me – now alongside that ambulance parking bay, I could feel a heaviness which was not there in my body – how would I even manage all the way into the hospital – even if Inno and Zeph would hold me by the shoulders side by side, would I make it.....?

And while in this endless thought, suddenly my medical friend returned – Israel, his name of course, was splendid – the wheelchair he wheeled along seemed an aeroplane when I saw it in my eyes, and I was light with peace of mind again. Interestingly I had lightning-strength to get 'me' over onto it, and without need of anyone's hand – at least someone had ensured its wheel-brake was on – in we entered into casualty – nice lady-doctor we meet.

Lockdown security rules

I suppose, like all other governments worldwide, ours would not be left out of making new policies in this special corona virus era. Indeed the new rule: 'every potential admission had to see the patient obtain a COVID TEST'

Blessing or no blessing, my result would only come out on Day 4 – Africa! What would this mean, wait and see!

The young lady doctor, explained in the most gentle way, did the nasopharyngeal test in the most careful way, finished her procedures for admission as earliest as she could (but mind you, arrival at Casualty was about 7pm, and the ward-bed received my back at 10pm – the cold of the night ensured my awakened state, and I don't believe I could be mistaken here a jot!). I thanked her with my heart. The wheelchair, even without an engine, in my childlike mind, I think it started it running, and down the long alley, up to the Western end, and fortunately an elevator we found working, and electricity full-time available (indeed by the grace of God – how would I have been lifted up the stairway?).

Somehow I don't recall if at all there was any activity at the Ward's nurses' station – whether the chilling numbness of the night stole it all – but here comes the moment of hopping on to the beautiful and promisingly warm bed – only the Corner house would have been extra-generous with a hot-water bottle (far from it that I would ever imagine asking for one!). And I knew one procedure soon coming – my dear friend would have to prick me – a drip had since been needed up badly!

The drip and first anti-Malaria injection – the stat dose

Something quite interesting, at least to me – I don't mind pricking myself, remember I would draw my own blood – yet my skin is not so friendly to even the prick from a friend – and unfortunately Israel's first was a miss, and he insisted as I twisted the face of my heart and hid my countenance in order not to bother my closest medical pal – fortunately, a good and sound doctor as he is – soon the next thing is to acknowledge his failure, and that much he did with a sorry I never doubt its genuineness. Then it was, that I realized that, my brilliant venous structure, was now collapsed and sort of sucked-in! Israel confirmed my dehydration – I think, from 4pm back home, to effective admission at 10pm at the hospital, the six hours of drinking or eating nothing, certainly added to the worst. Fortunately the second attempt hit the bore, and nowhere near the tendon this time. I was to remove the blood-restraining cotton wool strapped on the failure-site after some moments – I didn't wait long.

Normal saline ran in fast, I remember the doctor's command to the nurse, and one pack ran in, I realize, whilst Israel was still present by the bed side. Another one, he had to leave running, but the stat dose I trust he did it himself, of Artmether injection, to his friend who wouldn't take orally due to severity of complications of illness – and as I felt it in at the initial moment, I think I was to hear only his 'Goodnight' next, and he left, never tired due to LOVE, indeed the LOVE of God that found his soul!

The night of violation of the hygiene principle

On this first night, drips ran in initially fast as already mentioned, to be later-on regulated, and everything was under watchful eyes and done in time. Somewhere before sunrise the following day, a second anti-Malarial injection was given, I didn't quite feel it or notice it though.

The early hours of my bedtime were met with a different character all together in my adult-lifetime – those drips had truly been filling, and my reins were responding, filtering and making and sending down urine to my bladder. The latter could not handle the speed, and so I would strangely be in a dreamy state about it, stand by the edge of the bed in a most unusual way – the unfortunate end-result, I could fill the warmth of the liquid which never 'bathed' me before in adult-life. Then I would get onto the bed again, forget it all till the cycle would return to that point once again. I don't know if this happened about three times before a nurse, possibly noticed it. For at some time in the early morning hours, I observed a urine pot, lying flat upon a chair pushed to the edge of the bed. From this hour I was to know for certain what I would be doing, even went to the toilet alone to empty a full pot before sunrise. But somehow by sunrise, I took not notice of my wet bed, at least till the next morning as shall be revealed in more detail. The day went with deeper enjoyable sleep till I would be awakened for the injection, or for food which I was to always surprise the benevolent servers by touching nothing till 4 days lapsed. Indeed I ate no hospital food or any other, and my involuntary total fast lasted till my fourth day of admission.

Saturday the second day was not really full of stupor-like states, but I enjoyed those long periods of sleep. Innocent came in early to see me, with his wide smile I enjoyed so much – he stayed in quite long, but due to the deep enjoyable sleep, I wasn't to miss him much after he left.

I've almost forgotten to mention that earliest of morning visit, by my dedicated medical friend – Israel – must have been before 6am and I heard the door open with 'authority' – his big smile, commented on the temperature coming down – happy with what the two stat-doses had done so far – some instructions to the nurse who followed in, as I would be stolen by deep snaps.

And honest like him, before he goes out, he tells me frankly and straight: 'Wizzy – remember to mind your oral care!'

A while after he left when I reawakened, I checked my face in a mirror – horrible – a band of bloody stuck mucus firmly fixed upon my upper and lower front set of teeth! Not removable with water alone. Back to bed – a timely phone call – our remarkable Shepherd – Pastor – 'anything you need me to bring you?' he goes, and I receive with an apt request: 'a small towel and a toothbrush'.

Inno was to bring our own company's tooth-cleanser and liquid-soap, and Israel's concern would be well-met, but more accomplished on Sunday morning.

Saturday night went faster, with greater consciousness at the voiding wakes – and no spilling from myself or from the urine-pot. But the sleep episodes were deep, as I repaid the debt of about 6 weeks of slow-growing illness prior to hospital admission. A brilliant Sunday morning arrives and I'm as wide awake as is the sun's radiance by the wide window! Before I close here to go on to a lovely Sunday, let me confirm, that Pastor did faithfully bring the towel and the toothbrush, while Inno brought the soap and yet another pair of toothbrushes.

Here we are – Sunny Sunday!

The sun was smiling, and I could smile now too. But a single problem I had. Realization indeed occurred, that there was a stench of urine from my blankets, growing in intensity.

What a Sunday, blessed with some Nightingale pattern of nurses, so gentle, not only willing to help, but indeed practically and capably helpful. One of them entered, and I explained how in the dreamy state of the height of illness upon admission, my bed was in a mess with typical stench of fermenting urine. She was compassionate. She asked if I had bathed, and was shocked upon my 'No' to find that the out-going Night-staff had not even brought me water for bathing (for it is not a surprise to find no water on the wards, let-alone hot water – it has to be brought in a small dish).

Water was made ready for my bath – and I bathed my body like mine – each time surprised to feel the strength coming too. Upon finishing, I realized my bed was fresh and warm with ironed linen again. If only God may bless those sisters in multiple times, whom I cannot locate or recognize so easily now. Dr Israel was soon to pass by and was happy to see me sitting in a couch by the window – and he emphasized: Chris (physician), is going to visit today – I was glad I was neat and my bed was clean too. Israel had hailed when he saw me in the armchair: 'This is the Wiz I know!'

To this day I don't know how I shall pay best these two for a whole-hearted job they did without reservation upon their own. Indeed Chris arrived in with his old smile, looking quite young – and I couldn't hold my spontaneous shout: 'Ah Chris!'

He showed to be a master of his art and job – a quick objective assessment, as I listen to his briefings with the ward-round nurse, and soon he was satisfied – he waved me good-bye, and knowing how busy they are, as I would have been also, I wouldn't express how I missed having a few more seconds with him – and off, he waved his good-bye upon what I didn't realize then was to be his single and last visit. All this good, something, somehow would be lurking in the dark somewhere, in some way! My great God-fearing father had taught me – to always bank sound prayers in the times of good.

Innocent would soon arrive too, and he did – oh how I cherished his visits – enjoyable from start up to the end – and we would talk – face to face – brother to brother – no single hateful feeling – love greeting love – it was all so wonderful on the 'sunny' Sunday.

One concern upon Innocent's remark growing stronger: *'Mukoma'*, as he lovingly and respectfully addressed me in the vernacular, *'this is Day 3 and you haven't eaten anything!?'*, trying even to persuade me to take some of our company's cereal-fruit juice of which he had brought plenty of bottles into the ward-fridge – yet my appetite was shut, even though this was a juice 'tailored' to my tongue!

At some point not so far from that moment I made another 'discovery' – which I would have shined with like a child – saliva! Saliva? I was so worried it might never come again, and it would be very ominous! I made a display on my tongue to Inno of the spittle and all of us were happy in thankfulness to God. Inno's persuasions insisted that I make a solemn promise of when to eat, and I reinforced the fish dish. This my mother was going to bring on the morrow, and as though prophetic, I had promised everyone that this would be my first meal. Wait until the day after Sunday, and you shall know for certain it did happen.

The nurses were to surprise us, amidst our happiness, that Visiting Hour had lapsed by at least an hour, and I had to sadly miss Inno – I needed him so much for that day, wish they would allow him till dusk. Anyone who's been on the wards, no matter what kind of warding-in, knows the value of a visit from a true loved-one.

Sunday night had a team so contrary to afternoon's blessing. I even refuted to have my blood sugar checked by them – one of them had showed 'savage' characteristics upon pricking me on a previous night.

The night before the day

This was a special night to me. I expected great changes overnight so that my mother would see me having made strides in recovery. Yes, Mum, indeed she was coming on the morrow. And I had ordered local-rice and bottle fish-steaks. She knew how to prepare it the way I loved it. And I was expectant, I literally could taste the fish in my mouth. I wasn't quite sure about the rice, but when all would ask me if I would surely eat after a 4 day fast, I promised solemnly on the fish – the rice, somehow, I could no longer be that sure. I could see my mother, picture her and even imagine her elegant and respectful attire.

Let me tell something about my mother; you can tell I love her, and truly deeply. It dates back to an interesting background of bonding too. During my 11years of Epilepsy, we would cry together, pray together, sing together, travel and hunt for medicines together, do some fomentations together, eat and drink together (no beer for us of course). We believed together, that one day I would heal. And interestingly we shared this thing about caregiving with regards to my career. Thank God, He healed me a great four years before my entrance into the medical school in 1988. This is the mother who would see me tomorrow, and I would see her too, having been carried to the hospital in her absence. And the night was great, at least it was normal. The morning would be ominous, but nice, because of Mum – but the afternoon was not, indeed the 'viral' corruption would begin to surface.

The night went fast and my bath was thorough – selected my best raiment for meeting Mum – and sat by the wide window to bath in sun-rays. But something was strange of the night to show too in the morning. No one cared about my drips and the IV meds. And the last vaco-litre could have dripped in from the time of my sleep but to have no replacements. I was expectant but the thought of Mum erased the memory to remind the nursing team of the drip. After all, how many were to come into my room from then on.

Inno would have been the first one to come, but this morning he was on duty, manning our herbal-food shop at the nearby shopping centre.

Not long, our Isheanesu would stroll in with his confident steps upon favourite brilliant soft-stepping tuckies. We affectionately call him Anesu or by syllable-pronunciation Ane, as I welcomed him about 1000hrs. I knew him and Zeph had brought Mum, which he confirmed – a few seconds we are by the nurses' station – some oddest of odd behavior to literally push me back into the ward – but we read not the lines underneath the message, only to learn on the morrow. I straight way sought to see the matron, who might have read my eyes before my countenance, that

15

I was going to see my old lady, downstairs on the car, and never allow her to come upstairs. And the matron mumbled a funny phrase, which though audible, allowed no place of translation or consideration for the moment: 'Oh, this one, I've got his results (patting her breast area as though whatsoever she meant, was in her bra), I know them, he can go downstairs!' The aisle was short to reach the stairs, hand gripping hand for my giddiness and possibly lightheadedness. The stairs a bit of some labor – hop we lightly come off the last stair – soon out through the aluminium double glass door facing the finalists' medical residence. There's the Familia only 10metres away – expecting Mum's smile – oh, why it never crossed my mind she could actually cry! Indeed she had read my mal-balance, no matter how I tried to hide it. Greetings in the formal and traditional way yes, but not many seconds to pass before the bowl of rice and soup was on my laps. Fish is the 'chicken' of our family! Mum naturally doesn't take chicken. So we were saved so much from the GMO's. I had to leave some for the hours to come, not knowing they were going to be so harsh and terrible – the COVID era – 'corrupt' virus era!

That Afternoon of the clear-cut 'aura'

One thing to mention before I carry on – they did not bring James my 11+year old son on the trip – had been hoping to see him too – lockdown emphasizes distancing and it has affected the sitting/carrying capacity of smaller cars, especially sedans like ours. I understood the explanation and immediately put the thought of missing him aside.

Now the departure left me alone and lonely. And on this day too I missed the conversations with Inno.

Something of this 'drought' could have led me to go out about 1600hrs to just have a walk along the corridor may be to relieve this aloneness and loneliness – I think the nurses' station was empty, lest they would have jumped on me to stop me and pack me back again into the 'gaol'!

The telephone!

Yes, it was the matron, she was on the telephone, and her words were loud and clear and precise: '*Oh my dear, eeeeh! Yes! That doctor! Yes the one who was admitted with a positive test for Malaria. His results for COVID have eventually been reported to be* **POSITIVE***; and now I don't know what to do about the children – it's unfortunate you were here with them visiting, you know!'*

I was exactly by her wide open door, listening, and frozen but mind-active, as I watched her with her face and long hair down, really indulging herself in the telephone conversation. You would guess, from her age, she was probably talking to a beloved daughter, and was concerned about her grandchildren – who could have paid a visit along with their mother to see their granny the matron.

Before she finished, I receded my steps, quit the reaching of the corridor-end, and went back straight to the ward, reached my door handle, went right back in, closed firmly, and for some time I don't think any seat, chair or bed knew my buttocks or my back. The nurses station – when I passed by it – no – I don't believe any nurse was back there yet. I had heard the conversation which (according to the matron) I was not to hear – but why did God make me hear it at this stage.

It was dusk soon, the beauty of daylight had been stolen. The moon, even if it was to shine, this was town – the lights flood and override the mind – useless to look through the window, unlike back in our rural home where the curtain-less open louver reveals to heal a longing mother, missing and seeking the soul of a dear husband working in a far land.

All the same, God had found it sound in his undoubted wisdom to furnish and alert me before the two visitors at midnight.

The puzzle is clear and flowing!

There are crossword puzzle lovers and possibly even addicts – but one of what I would call: **good addictions,** especially for a child learning with a future to converse and link in the world at large.

Impossible would it seem at first, especially to a starter. But the regular fan, one word, then the second also vertical, a third and fourth horizontal, even the fifth and sixth with some crossing and linking – and the hinting, the supposition, the prediction and the sound guessing begin to come. Soon everything flows smoothly to hit the end. It's done.

My friends and family know this to be my original: 'Some complex, hard to understand, or some unbefitting message or word or information, even some unfitting and puzzling situation – put on the shelf – 'tomorrow' it shall show – ripened or rotten – liquidized or sublimed – truth or lie – sound or trash – godly or ungodly – and the Lord blesses such an attitude of faith and prayer while you wait upon him.

Now the unchanged drips, the lack of attention, dried up nurses' visits, the stopped medicines (but this one was an immediate puzzle – obviously too inhumane to accept anywhere in the medical and nursing world!), the ward turned prison, the disdain and the hate on me – as though I was a man turned dog – as though someone would spit me in the face to show me the way back into the 'jail'!

And I sat on the chair, sipping and breathing in the cold, the bed became as though one, an adulterer, had just been caught and convicted on. Soon it was an hour before midnight. Forgot the beautiful fish altogether – yet plenty of it remained in the bowl in the fridge, with the rice untouched. I wished they would talk to me. I wasn't afraid. But I needed to be out any moment. The 'boys' would never be 'faraway' in distance or in time – it would be an easy mission for them. But I was, had not known and would never have guessed, going to be restrained till 5pm the following day before starting on the way back home.

Mercy department had closed. Security department had taken over. No one remembered the sufferer with Malaria, except in description. All perceived a monster coughing, drooling, sneezing and wee-weeing COVID 19. And only tomorrow would I know it, that when you would be 5metres within their reach, a COVID-diarrhea's pungent diffusion would be blowing them away, as they would shout at you in disgust.

Silence broken

A knock and an entry – an old fashioned lady you would think, but no, it was some improvised dressing for COVID!

A guard had been sent me, I knew straightway from her weird words – 'I have been assigned to you, hear whatever help you may need and assist you on this night!'

The words cut me – but I had to be kind, and I think by the beginning of the morning I had earned my first convert – convert from a 'COVeeD'!

Hardly an hour, a familiar lady came in – the devoted lady-casualty officer. She remained her nice self. Not mincing her words and without delay, she said the story, full of concern and compassion. She mentioned the responsible doctors, who were in a meeting which never seemed to end downstairs, and I didn't know that, the name which kept on coming, was the retired colonel who would be on the money-driven mission to be visiting me on surveillance and investigation – not for love or treatment – but for 'security' – with zeal and fuel in him and his partner even to arrive at night for the sake of money claims at the end of day.

The young lady-doctor, did all she could, genuinely to counsel and to advise. Only they could not help me with a phone charger (as my friends had kept on forgetting mine), whether genuinely or deliberately. And this reminds me, one episode I had forgotten in that afternoon of the matron's phone aura: I went to the nurses station to ask them to help me charge my phone – and I was literally scoffed at – another hard puzzle-breaker to fit some missing unfilled part.

The lady doctor would soon leave with nice parting words and well-wishing (to a bat-bitten earlobe). Soon she was to leave, together with the fat lady! Wonder who had planned the order of their coming?! She tried to persuade me to go back to sleep, but I firmly told them, I would rather remain seated in the armchair till morning. Little did they know, and would never realize that within an hour, COLD would drive and shove me into the linen, but with all my clothes (except footwear for sure – I was still sane), till the entire bed guarded the warmth from this extra-warm-blooded mammal, and somehow sound sleep was broken as morning was broken. It had been a mind-resting sleep of possibly 5 hours. The fat lady seemed to help in the daybreak – I think she must have knocked – was bringing bath water next, she advised – that little hot 'aliquot', I had since grown to love and enjoy, never thinking of our plentiful solar-heated showering amounts back home.

The last day in prison-tal? Jail-tal? Gaol-tal?

A single test result, not even a diagnosis, for a positive test has to be evaluated in the context of the entire condition, situation or state – yes – I had never realized such a single positive test, more so as an incidental finding could change a hospitality centre into an imprisonment centre! And all care for humanity seemed lost. I had now entered the second day without any treatment for the unfinished Malaria course – more than 24hours without a drip now, and on the second day, till I would leave hospital, no one would care a tittle about the Artemesinine/Lumafantrine tablets that were supposed to take over from the IV Artmether injection. Dear doctor, if I was your son, your brother, your father – what if the plasmodium was still reigning and residing in hidden corners – wasn't there a danger of creating resistance to medication – where is the kindness gone – have the medical personnel escaped and their places taken over by jailers, prison guards or any other security officers. The latter sounded more of a favorable term – there was a new set of medical officers, indeed COVID security officers, and the power of the true caregivers was also crushed and squashed beneath their own self isolation in the lockdown. And the new team of authority, would never care what treatments or stage of therapy one was on, the evidence is there, and not only above, but more to come as the account proceeds to demonstrate the impact of corruption of virology upon humanity.

This security team, has given me nothing to this day except:

1. Greetings in hypocritical grins
2. Disdain
3. False promises amid procrastinations and postponement of visits when dates are due for samples
4. Threats, some of them corruption-driven if not only to show the venomous glands behind fangs that make the victim irk in helplessness
5. Injuries – from the invasive procedures, with a range of affections from risks like paranasal sinus inflammations up to carvenous sinus thrombosis and complicated relational states

6. Low esteem and defamations of all sorts
7. Exacerbation of your aloneness and loneliness especially when seeking to frustrate for corrupt COVID gains
8. Stigmatization and all the segregation that comes with it – if the victim is not careful or has no way of disposing the 'wastes' from this end, it may subtract value from their life and livelihoods
9. Hunger and lack and want of essentials in life
10. No good, No virtue

Your own, you have to love despite.......

Your very-very own still love you, and there is nothing they can do, they can't help themselves – and somehow God has helped them to see crystal-clearly, what is there and what is imagined, what is really proven versus suppositions, what motives and attitudes reign in the COVID action team (that one to quickly dissolve and disappear when the real phenomena of the disease in its full phenotypic characteristics strikes to that extent of not even entertaining the testing centres – for all cowards, as I've previously hinted, will run away and hide, if not perish).

Now reality: One's own have always nursed and cared for their own in past scourges since time immemorial. You have to give them food to eat, something to drink, water to bath, fresh air, a clean environment and a good toilet facility if not even consistently help them to use it functionally fully to real relief and a cleansed state. When you truly analyze these things, then a wise one will take note: Better to pray hard that the situation in the West, North and East is stayed from even coming down to Africa! For who would indeed under our culture ever live without to mind his own? If you carelessly think: 'Far from it!', think about your helpless child, your mother who has cared for you to the reminders of Mother's Day – imagine what it would take for you to be angry at them in serious suffering, and more so, innocently! Would you in reality fly away? At least for now, the airlines are grounded – where will you go?

Let us tell each other the truth here: hygiene and safety remain the rule – and if this is done with love and longsuffering – the inert and the active defense lines will build frontline aiders a more securely reliable protective and safety barrier. Best resisters build defense from within! Such will live, not by chance. And with God's love, they have remained always, nothing short of the Pilot Psalm – Psalm 91!

Kicked out into the hands of my own

In our vernacular, we've got a famous proverb of reminiscent meaningfulness: *'Kukava datya watoriyambutsa'*

Given an expounded translation, it would open up this way: '*You might think you've* **kicked a frog away** *into its misery, when in actual fact, as mercy would have it, you've enabled its* **cross-over** *unto sound safety and secure prosperity'*

Shame, it's of terrible depravity to be kicked, but being kicked off and lobbed over to be grabbed into the hands of loved ones, I should thank God ten thousand of times, given the capacity.

Lets pip into the beginning of the next chapter – and see how our own receive, no matter how rejected and repelled we may be! **Let Love be without dissimulation** (Romans 12v9) is what meant to be home again. And I was to have mercy of being received into such a home again.

CHAPTER THREE

DISCHARGE

Separation beyond segregation

The discharge influenced by hatred yet effected by love

Loving doctors did the discharge summary and wrote the prescription for my continuation with the oral tablets for Malaria. This was a good deal and perfect deed to cover the nursing head on discontinuing the injectables and the IV fluids, and it all appeared she must have pushed for that discharge. But then she would have explained to me by right – nothing was done; and she and the new doctors (the security team), should have ensured my continuation with the orals, but for two days they were quiet, with no concern whatsoever. What an ugly separation of hate! Segregation beyond highest degrees of quarantine! Two days of no medicine at all – what will stop any loved and reasonable one from asking: 'Why? Did they want to kill you?'

I've posed this act to the responsible 'security docs', and they have passed a casual 'sorry'. Reader, what do you think?

Stay-in 'breathlessness' makes me seek fresh air, and I leave the ward forever

Without medication two days, and without any explanation why, I felt a hypoxia within the drives of my mind! Whatsoever was happening outside this past hour of the afternoon? Where were my own loved ones?

23

On this day have they stayed them from coming in and left me to ponder the explanation. I didn't have enough air in the room to conjure adequate thoughts on alternative plans to relieve the sphincters of my brains in this position. It is terrible when others do unto you what they would never love to be done unto themselves. I was later to ask one male nurse while upon the stairs as he distanced himself 5metres higher up: 'What's a colleague, am I a colleague, is this the way you would treat/handle a colleague?' He was thoughtful, and he held his tongue and sealed his vocal chords.

Now let me tell you what I did, thoughtlessly or thoughtfully, but the truth is, I couldn't handle the pressure any longer – diagnosis = Malaria, and two days lapsing without medication, no explanation; my own not around for visiting hour and no explanation in the after-hours!?

I had since packed all my items in plastic bags in the morning, in fact, like dirty rags and linen with COVID. But myself, I was dressed neatly, though great strain of un-wellness and psychosocial imbalance distorted my countenance like one with a splitting headache akin to cerebral irritation – yet I had no headache.

'Don't come out, stay inside!' The nurse at the nurses station shouted, I did not care her presence. And she shouted, no 'please' in her statements, rather it was as though she was addressing a dog. Now past that matron's office, with nothing in my hands, all plastic bags left inside after I slithered past the half-open door that I had to close again gently. Full, I noticed, was the matron's office. They all saw me past as I reached out to Inno by the office right next to the stairs – I supposed the clerk's, for statements and payments, and I was right. The matron's cheeky nursing team, initially dead silent, began to literally bark themselves (positions may change so easily), the moment I started down the stairs after whispering with Inno. I stopped amid the stairs to answer them, but each one of them with his or her loudest yell, how would they hear me – a brief moment, maybe the male nurse silenced them to give an ear to this 'COVeeD dog', and all I said: 'I just want to go downstairs to our car, the familia you see a minute away, and rest, and breathe different air.' He heard it, but his reasoning I couldn't bear. Their yelling as I proceeded step by step, was caught like a netball by the guards who blocked the stairway exit with hospital food-carriages (if that's what they call those wheeled cages hooked upon each other like a train). I lay myself down upon the stair before the last step – now the male nurse seemed to hear me well – he went upstairs and came up with their first reasonable answer and act – the 'trucking-gate' had to be opened, to the dismay of many, even the 'vigilant' guard who rhetorically asked the air: 'Wakunda? Wakunda?' meaning 'Has he won? Has he won?', and within seconds I lay myself on the rear couch of our Familia. My body sucked in all the westerly sweet sun with gladness felt entirely. I breathed well in the presence of those who never rejected me, those I should have given tonnes and tonnes of COVID well before I had come to the hospital – but to this day, as I have said before – not a single person in my contact-tracing under their surveillance program has tested positive for the disease.

We are yet to officially and legally prove that a professional from the local/home-area hospital must have initiated hate messages from his phone which littered my name into the public in menacing words, phrases and sentences unto wretched defamation. We have all wondered why, and for the sake of the medical community, we feel it has to be looked into.

The officials in Harare said they had handed us to our resident medical community, recently 'converted' into security officers because of my 'contraction' (they sounded sure to say or vow).

Nearby our rural home they claimed, and would say they would phone us, even till about 5pm – and would not allow us to drive an inch from the central hospital, even when we reasoned about buying the pharmaceutical drugs at a nearby chemist – the very treatment that was ceased for two days – we didn't understand it! Cruelty? But why? We were to discover more undoubted hatred and obvious hateful perpetrations, that no Public Health Act or law would be claimed to have sanctioned! Where on earth would one accept such a lie? For one officer of the health sector, claimed: 'All I'm doing is in accordance with the Public Health Act!' We wish God to have this officer proven wrong.

Between 4 and 5pm, let me say this before leaving this section, they reported to be evaluating our Garden Centre and proposed Corner house for my isolation – it is strange, we hear they did that and disinfected the room with its restrooms and toilet pan around 10am, and were never back in the garden. Yet they delayed us telling us as though they were actually busy in the garden around 4-5pm? A type of 'diplomacy'? Only acceptable in our realm if it's labelled a 'COVID-type diplomatic allowable strategy'!

Night travel

My constant pleading fell on deaf ears – 'It will be more reasonable if you enable me to travel during daylight.' I was a rat and a constant irritant to them – they seemed to have that desire to make me feel the bad end to its very extreme. And for some time, I think they counted their scores and tallied for themselves without the approval of the Just Umpire, thought they were winning, littered more hate Whatsapp messages, whose effect hit us upon our nocturnal arrival, receiving even scornful messages – and they most probably thought the damage had been done to kill and to destroy everything. But such thinking for professionals, the Heavens would only consider most foolish. In a world whereby one is loved by many for their life-saving work, that population is good and makes no mistakes at diagnosing hate messages especially stemming from jealous on progressive work/mission in rivalry. We hadn't an idea of their evil rivalry, but events do bring them to surface. Only God would rescue us. We needed to pray.

Travel and Arrival

This journey itself, seemed not exciting. Even the combustion chambers of the engine could have felt the risk of the coldness to quench the vehicle to a stop. We had dropped Inno by Epworth turnoff to catch some lifts to his family; we proceeded only as two, Zeph and myself. I was not in so much a state to hear him. He sped well. No hassle with the police. Who would love to tarry long with a 'COVeeD' anyway? Once they saw me the signal was to proceed. First stop was Mum's place, officially to drop off garments for the washing machine, but socially: 'How on earth would I get into self-isolation without seeing my Mum?'

After a face-to-face 'goodnight' that would last a while for Mum till another direct interaction, we left for the garden. Zeph would not be delayed now. It would be unreasonable. The night was getting deeper and darker.

The reunion with my friends, or my sons, my beloved ones – it was sweet and great – and our Lord had a new experience of an even higher level of love for us all. Paul of old: Romans 8v31

Who can separate us from the love of God?

No one, nothing, shall separate us?

And the scripture and even the song goes as if there is no stopping! I was welcomed back to the family which I should have given that alleged COVID of the test, yet I was not to transmit it up to this day 21-5-2020. And the first check test has been negative, the second check test with a story to come, results shall be out tomorrow. If all contacts remain negative, then what strange event to make this second one positive – it would be strangest of the strange indeed. Best – let's wait for tomorrow, in this world of the 'security' officers – medical officers have been put to sleep!

CHAPTER FOUR

───── ✑ ─────

DEFINITION

Reality of COVID in the light

Every doctor, who is a true caregiver and not just a certificate-holder, when a new condition dawns, he is instinctively switched into careful observation – to match what is described of a pestilence, whether it is truly a pandemic if reported so, or its affecting one race or tribe more than the other, comparing too the patterns of illness coming from different areas with that question: WHY THE DIFFERENCE?

If first cases are reported in his region, he's alert to analyze if the condition is presenting pure without other associated conditions, who is susceptible, what other conditions may seem to predispose victims to the new condition?!

He is careful – studies the presentation well, not just the test and test-results. He is naturally and usefully interested in the features of the illness clinically besides the international test – for at the end of the day, there ought to be a way of distinguishing with reasonable specificity that separates the disease without mistaken diagnosis/labelling, even before the test is done. And the earlier the defining of things from the surface and earliest stages, the better – for it is known that good doctors usually make 70% of their diagnosis from clinical assessment alone (history & examination) before much investigation, some of which may be dangerously invasive.

At this stage, I have got to state my wish:

I wish a test is devised soon for asymptomatic cases in the 'COVID' screen program, which doesn't put thousands of health individuals at the risk of the _invasive_ access to their sinuses, both the para-nasal air sinuses and the cavernous sinus, as I have witnessed with the nasopharyngeal swab.

And I quickly return to our dedicated and talented doctor. It has been said by some wise one in the field of medicine: 'The gift of a doctor is best defined on a field-visit into a rural/village community expanse'

Truly, there is no X-ray or scan there – where there's no blood test access – no sputum, urine, stool specimen for laboratory analysis there.

And the gifted practitioner defines illness patterns and separates them cost effectively for very necessary investigation and apt one most of the time, should such be really necessary to help the sufferer, and always remembers **to do no harm first.**

This latter we shall always have to remember in relation to our 'COVID' story in the African nations, where company workers risk being screened with terrible invasive access to their special cavities, yet without real illness patterns of COVID showing within our communities – what is going to be the impact of these invasive procedures, not in the hands of trained ENTs, but, 'girls and boys' digging for money in the program, and they are excited when they throw the swab-stick like a spear to hit the mucosa, may be twist it with as much strength as they can that they don't miss any bit of positive diagnosis?

Our cautious doctor also is wary, where the investigative kits have come from - which country or nation – and seeks to know what population-types where involved in the calibration of the test kits – he wishes calibration was effected for his own communities before such surveillance tools are used – and tries to guard against false positives – ensuring retesting soon after a co-existing condition is cleared.

The hallmark of the matter here is: Where real disease is rampant as in the West, North and East, tests will confirm what the community and the doctors are already seeing in illness pattern. Whereas Southerly down Africa, the adopted screening method, without experience, due to lack of existence of real illness pattern, dangerous reality of defining unrealistic and non-existing ailment – the consequent: the public may suffer complications at the hands of money-mongers.

One should go to the public or private centres of testing, and observe the attitude and actions of staff there – whom I have always told:
'Sure, my sisters and brothers, better make money now and enjoy, lest the real thing is here early'
Because the truth is, when the patterns that lead to death really surface in Africa, this cowardish and noisy 'frontline pattern of crew' flees and/or disappears altogether. They are the 'gold panners' along innocent rivers that for years were flowing naturally without any damage. And the unpredicted impact after invasion is regrettable. Today I personally suffer a para-nasal **sinusitis** that I only hope its impact will not last the rest of my lifetime! You shall indeed hear more about this.

What is 'COVID' in our setting?

The 'medical community' have a lot of influence in how the public will define an illness, based on various factors: their attitudes, their motives, their prowess, their ignorance, their integrity, their patriotism and philanthropy or lack thereof, their alertness, their guard against intruders and destructive foreign materials or even policies, their lack of care due to not understanding the value of their populations and ecosystems, their love of money and tendency to corruption etc.

Hear this: the local officer in charge of health, in charge of a district-expanse reaches the Garden Centre gate and spits these words at my 11year old son James: *'Mudhara wako akuudza here kuti arohwa neCOVID?'* literally meaning 'Has your old-man told you that he's been struck with COVID?'
(When I sent an sms to this officer's phone to find out: **Why?** he replied, 'Because I wanted him to open the gate for me....' His answer shocked me! I enquired by sms because I wanted the record)
Tino who was there by the gate informed me, they had trouble comforting James who continued in sobs for a long period (even the officer

testified in his reply sms, that there was a certain guy with James by the gate at his telling him the above words).

Also hear this one: a team packed in a land-cruiser Toyota alights and enters my mother's homestead and one of them shouts at her as they just enter the gate: 'Mwana wenyu abatwa neCOVID!' closest in meaning: 'Your son has been hit by COVID!'

Now, Mum, currently 75years old, is a retired trained primary school teacher who served, teaching in the kindergarten for 42years in various schools in our nation of Zimbabwe. You should hear how she felt, in her brief account at the end-pages.

And hate messages on the Whatsapp platform stated and claimed the name of the officer in health, who had spread the messages!

It is useful to exonerate this officer for the sake of the future of medical ethics, officially via the Police Charge Office, so that the messages are proven to have not come from his phone. And to prove him a clean ethical officer who doesn't mess up with names as he observes confidentiality. He should be happy to have his name freed from the local community's pointing-of-fingers at him as the source of the initial hate-messages.

Why? What am I driving at by all this: The public at large, has a definition of an illness/COVID, in accordance with how the medical community portrays or conveys that definition to it.

And the stigma is ignited, then bellowed upon in blasts of mockery, nicknames, despise, hatred, misjudgments, distrust, and even up to the height of persecutions in the cloud of segregation created by corrupt 'frontline' mongers.

Example – when the community grips the wrong definition

There is a 70year old lady who lives naturally like us, has worked in our Natures' Food Haven (NFH) Project, four days per week for the past 7+years, and walks 4km from her homestead where she looks after her grandchildren, many of them **orphans**, herself being a **widow** for more than ten years now. She has an elder sister whose homestead is within a kilometer from our NFH Garden Centre, and the two of them take turns to look after their old mother, who is possibly 100+years, no longer walking and requiring assistance in a number of day to day issues of living.

This Granny, famously addressed 'Gogo' in the garden, was blatantly told not to fetch water from the borehole – 'in order not to give us your COVID which you have obtained from your 'Gwatidzo'!'

In strategy, for some time, she has had to rise up in the wee-hours of the morning to fetch water and avoid serious consequences of such segregation – being a very peaceful elderly lady amongst her own – now no one sees all that today.

You shall get a chance to listen to her own story-telling at the end pages.

The comment of a dull certificate-holder

One friend and medical colleague, phoned to enquire on me when I was now back home a few days post discharge – and said:

'Your Malaria must have been serious due to COVID....'

I shut his mouth:

'You know W, I have not suffered any illness related to COVID 19, before admission with Malaria, during the admission or even post admission – that was an incidental finding of a positive test, and you as a medical professional, I expect you to comprehend that perfectly well!'

He had not been an intelligent one ever amongst our class, but he managed to find a niche in an apt specialty somehow quite befitting his mind.

He apologized and would soon have to make his call shorter. My two doctors on the ward, the physician and the surgeon were careful and have professionally reasoned and figured out the chances of real COVID disease remote from my situation. Potentially false positives do exist, and coward COVID security officers do detect them and pursue them (being sure of their safety) strongly and diligently for the sake of amassing sums of money from the usually internationally or local-donation sponsored programs. And they are ruthless, without any care – hence they can cut out a patient's original treatment altogether with no compassion to ensure the continuity means availed by the original medical doctors – rather 'imprisoning' the neo-labelled sufferer without any thought about his/her living.

False death message

On one night, the phone rang in the middle of the night, and there was a familiar voice of a concerned friend, not afraid, but to warn me of a false death message – he said it read:

'Dr Gwatidzo is now dead from COVID'

I thanked him and immediately warned all my co-workers and family members!

Had I passed on from Malaria, my intelligent colleagues who managed me unto 'revival', I can guess here, would never have accepted 13000 US dollars to put COVID 19 on the causes of that demise upon the death certificate. Have you not read dear reader? Aren't you following authentic news? That the above is indeed happening in the West to entice doctors to write COVID death certificates? Oh COVID corruption – what a scandal from 'birth' to 'death', from 'poor' to 'rich', from 'ignorance' to 'well-aware', from 'cot' to 'coffin', and from 'work' to 'lockdown'!

Dear Reader – can you read the puzzle?

And how can you read it well whilst in **lockdown** or **quarantine** – and they are busy in '*mining*' and *cashing*?

And they teach you '**social distancing**', whilst they are pairing in the most horrible acts of corruption?

Wonder if anyone is reading whilst in **isolation** – I'm writing this book whilst in an isolation that a cruel 'master' with a grudge has vowed an intention to extent to 6weeks in total – doesn't care if that will be healthy for my mind or well for my suffering and calling patients!

And I have warned this 'boss':

'Each time God shall hear the cry of my patients, the curse shall fall upon your head!'

Well – **ISOLATION** – may you take a glimpse of the title of the next chapter!

CHAPTER FIVE

———— ✑ ————

ISOLATION

Enabled is the hiding of the sins of 'actors'

I'm so happy to find you here dear Reader, and I'm sorry to have dwelt on the sad things too much – hopefully you are not discouraged – one of our great fathers influenced me:

'You may turn every challenge you meet in life into living business solutions'
(How? - By grace and by faith)

Let me tell you about the second day's morning in the garden with my two dear friends whom together with other wise ones, accepted me and never rejected me.

But before I begin, I should inform you of what happened in the hospital after I suddenly felt strongly missing them in late hours of the third night. My phone had now been always switched off as it was great labor to attend to its calls on me in all its electronic provisions, and this was my third night. I switched on the phone as soon as the memory of my loved ones was switched on by the Lord. And I phoned on Tino's line: Oh a happy snapshot moment, and New (as Tino affectionately short-named Newton) was by his side, and I'm still to ask them what they were talking about at that hour – otherwise I wouldn't have delayed in telling you – as for myself I had only the Lord. Could they have been talking about me, the culminating events unto my admission, themselves or whatever? Should these dear ones of mine tell me, and it's enjoyable, I shall give you a glimpse of taste at some distance ahead in your reading.

Our first morning in Bible-reading and Prayer on reunion

Now here we run:

Whilst in hospital, well before I knew of my kick-off discharge, The Lord gave me a scripture to breakfast upon with my young friends: II Kings 2 – **never to turn back – always in the good consistent and insistent spirit – like an Elisha – till the cloak is in your hand**

We feasted upon that word and the Lord was merciful as we gave our prayer. He has always been kind to us. Day after day, together, we have seen His care. After prayer, I informed my two friends how the Lord had given me the scripture whilst in hospital to share with them on our first Bible Reading & prayer session – they were happily amazed but not amused. The Lord who had brought me back has always showed himself to us in such wonderful ways – so we are never to forget him!

We had woken-up in the famous Round House, just that arrangement of three couches, as we had slept before I was removed to the hospital. I am allergic to most sprays and disinfectants. The Corner House had been sprayed by the local COVID team, and though we had done our own part to cleanse, I felt I would only lie there on the morrow. I even wonder who supplied those disinfectants to our nation – hope not an evil 'seed' of burdens of tomorrow for a continent relying on covetous foreigners' industry. Need to wake up!

I was home now, the sun rose and I could sit and bath in its extra-healing rays. I was where I was accepted, where I was loved, where I was wholeheartedly offered wholesome food. A goat had been given in thanksgiving by Eddie, our friend who goes into the distal rural corners and mountainous border-areas ordering super-organic goats for resale in the Capital. And Pastor had delivered it already exceptionally well-prepared in a cooler box just before I left for admission at the hospital – so I hadn't had a chance on it. After-all my appetite had distanced itself. Now I was back and my body remembered. Thank God my loved ones had left a generous share for my recovery. And in recuperation they would take turns to prepare a dish for me, sometimes Mum in the Town Centre and our Jemu (affectionate short-cut of James) would bring via a safe road through the hospital and through the village – even our own village. Then our traditional staple would be prepared by our adept New with Africa's amazing bulrush millet. The plate was mouth-watering and I would feel regains in recovery each single day, during this recuperating period.

But let us be careful here – a whiff of a bad-wind from someone on the table may turn the entire supper for weak ones into an empty night as they abandon their meal – and there are people so easily discouraged by whiffs of pungent winds in forms of noxious words from the enemy's windpipe!

Be it far from you to resign – get into fresh air and bath the memories away soonest! Whiffs of Tobias and Sanbalath, Nehemiah blew off with gusts of faith and confidence in The LORD. Get your fans right. See the whiff below. You may at times never be face to face with your persecutors, but a prayer away, has tuned the Heavens to bring the gush in an earthquake to dispel the enemy's strategy – but would God have to send the huge tremor for a whiff – he expects you to brush it aside in trust and 'crunch' the snake's mouth before the entire garden inhabitants are spoilt in their hearts!

I had the 'opportunity' today (22/5/2020) to hear the immediate neighbours calling loudly upon one another to my derision: *'How is the COVID?'*

And in turn the other family spokes-superior would reply: *'The COVID is just going round in circles around the homestead'*

I didn't care a jot – I knew where all this had rooted from – indeed from rotten systems not original and not tailored to our own culture – in Africa we risk copying to the danger of extinction like a vapor. At the hospital it had been worse and here at home there were the echoes. Some day we shall be on the 'tables' and on the unreachable Rock: **to teach them** in the Lord.

I enjoyed my recovery. The body was 'lazy' – but my soul was not. I was not yet my original self – yet my spirit was happy. And my return, The Lord lit the garden with it. Everyone was happy. Not one among the hands God blessed to help me, would translate any load as a bothering burden – the care has been glorious to this day – only the Sunny Sunday team of nurses at the hospital could match the love (if you dear Reader remember them). The Lord has been amongst us, and to this day the Devil has a 'dyspepsia'! (In the vernacular we would say – '*Satani wakasvotwa kwazvo!*'

We even ordered another goat, to be so well-done, by our team in our NFH methods and stages of preparation for optimum bioavailability of the prepared dishes – enabling full nutrient uptake and incorporation into the tissues and organ-systems.

And indeed, the emaciation has gone, the swollen ankles suddenly went unnoticed – being from the Anemia which I stated earlier and the tongue and hands are red again, the giddiness is gone and I can even run, the consistently added strength I have often demonstrated by pushing Ane when he is unwary, the sight is more than what I previously thought was my normal (take note of goat meat and eyesight dear Reader), the gut is now almost normal – stools come down in almost single soft but firm raw of long sausage, often a first, then a second column seconds later, may be a little tail last – so easy to push; the face is humbly handsome and responds to wash with lovely brilliance (yes, the face reveals a lot about recovery), plus, I feel I am a man again indeed!

Only one thing was disturbing, the coming of the 'gold panners'! In fact it wasn't about their coming but their attitudes. One local set accosted on their first and tried to set in chaos in our centre, taking as if it was their playground, even trying to shoot videos – fortunately a firm NFH patriot on our team stayed them – the following day I reprimanded that *young guy* who had to present himself for the next 13days (total of 14) as a **'gentleman',** on their opportunistic 'mission' to earn US dollars

Let me tell you something sacred here: We have always worked in places separated and dedicated specially to The Lord. No soccer or plays or dramas in our settings. We are as in 'our Father's Business', after our Lord. And we guard our places jealously in our hearts as Abraham effectively guarded his offering (Genesis 15). Vultures, even ravens, cannot be partakers! Our endeavor: ALL BE TO THE GLORY OF GOD! We will never want to take away God out of our services.

We deal with The Lord's nature-haven (Exodus 15v25 & I Kings 4v33) and we aren't witchdoctors. Come to our practice and our shop and you shall testify to others.

Take <u>not</u> heed of the scornful messages of a fellow African, jealousy of the well-packaged produce & services by one of his own, yet not seeking God's Wisdom in appreciating how his brother has not only been blessed for himself alone, but for the blessing of that seed of tomorrow in the loins of all, including that hate-diffusing brethren! (The latter passes not only whiffs of pungent discouraging gas, but even the poisonous 'sulfur' from his volcanic-cratered end!)

Then the 'duet' of officers on cruise in the COVID-program's land-cruiser, the elder one leading his first part on his own crafted song: 'My prowess of diplomacy' as he hails himself – maybe forgetful deliberately of my knowledge of his in-charge of the team that left me for two days without any medicines for slide-proven Malaria at the hospital! But as I never keep faults and defects but rather deal with them for correction and maintenance of functional standards, I told him, and his response – 'sorry', a dry 'diplomatic' sorry! And his tongue 'thinks' that is the end of it all! Jokes! God is there! And He can lead an exploration by men, to the protective benefit of others in the future.

They paid three visits. The first upon which they took samples of blood and sent to the lab, confirming absence of Malaria. Wonder what else they could have assayed on their part in relation to COVID (e.g. antibodies) in order to tally for more money claims.

Then, they came next and for the first invasion of theirs into my nasopharyngeal cavity, to eventually disturb my sinuses with infective-inflammation, which I trust by God's grace it shall be cleared completely – test-results took long to come, indeed very long. It is their attitude, incomprehensible motives and actions that are very questionable, when the results delay – you would be given an imaginary probability?!

Interestingly, before the swab was plunged in, they asked if I was okay, and my answer startled them: 'Unless if you are going to inoculate me – otherwise I've been recovering so well!'

A rumor went out too that there was a shortage of reagents, but it appeared the officers themselves were the epicenter of that same rumor, spreading it first to ears of cadres they thought were honey combs guarded by bees of a weaker disposition! 'COVID'! In Africa? We shall see. Let's go on!

Isolation, if one is not careful, may subject the victim to impositions – tests and measures may be exerted upon the labelled one as though without a choice to check the considerations possible – it would appear like there is absolutely no choice for the victim and they are afraid of being accused of 'not cooperating' or 'being stubborn', 'rule-breaking' or just labelled 'a fugitive'. When they are injured, they might suffer more harm at the hands of an incapable 'trainee' on the program, who has not mastered techniques, and is doing harm as with sinus problems! But this is a system like of security forces in a bush-war, and victims seemingly cannot report against the vice of these 'superiors' anywhere or in some way – and when it is actually discovered that indeed they are not immune to the law of safety of any individual, at times it is too late – the victim is very mutilated with complications or at times even dead.

I jump the event-line here, for I've got something to tell:
Of the pair that took the swab whilst I was in isolation, somehow I trusted capacity without thinking. Normally I would enquire about the person and find out whom he is, his qualifications, and where he did train and what he is currently doing. Interestingly the 'post-mortem' enquiry after this cadre damaged my para-nasal air sinuses, revealed that he was a post-grad student in the department for treating the insane – I began to think how much care he could have of me on his heart. For when I told the senior one of my terrible predicament, he arrogantly defended verbally:
'Even myself I've a bad feeling from my sinuses from this type of investigation'
And that was that, he had 'finished'. I had to phone the City Health boss when I learnt of the booked date for the two's intended visit for a second swab – I requested earnestly to go to a private lab instead, after elucidating my story of the sinuses – indeed the previous night with the rising chilly air of growing Winter's cold nights, I had not slept as my

sinuses were like freezer compartments with split or injured inner linings – I rolled and turned, meanwhile pressing a hot-water bottle from one area of the scalp and face on my right side, even dangerously in front of my eye, to cover the maxillary sinus well! The water bottle, soon to get cold, I had to reheat the kettle and refill, almost every 30 minutes; and so for about nine hours, I was awake!

It was on the following morning that my request saw me be driven to a private testing centre. It was a Wednesday and the results would come up in two days' time. Before leaving that COVID testing centre, I got a phone call, with concern from the other voice that 'I was missing' – upon which I didn't bother to apologize to about the missing-bit, but report that the sinusitis had gotten worse, and I had asked to have the test in a different setting – this was not so gullible to the travelers – I wouldn't know if they could still claim their money, but certainly not for swabbing me, for they would not. I wonder what was happening to poor peasants who didn't know anyone! A granny, widowed years back and covering her orphans with weak wings and poor feathers, how would they even tell the wrong that was done to them?

Due to innervation, my teeth on the right side became extremely sensitive – that electrical phenomena which blocked sleep and kept me all the night long! Antibiotics have only helped a little to this day 23-5-2020, herbals having complemented far-better – but I'm still to finish the course that my friend prescribed after persuading me.

I am to travel into town to meet the head of the program in three days' time, to discuss way forward with regard to work in respect of patients crying for our clinical services, as well as in respect of my psychosocial status – for the COVID 'security' elder one of the two, has proposed an extension of my self-isolation up to 6weeks! Revenge spirit? COVID-corruption – yes!

Now dear Reader – Quarantine 6 weeks – what questions come to your mind?

1. When did this isolation extension to cases begin and could the amended written policy be provided?
2. Is the extension-measure not officer-initiated to 'discipline' a sufferer; or it's genuinely on the strategy as new, or it can be a discretional measure in extreme of difficult situations – what difficult situation does two negative tests pose?
3. Is it possible to know how many people are under such protracted 'jail' term at the moment?
4. What forms of support are availed for someone in such a mind-boggling quarantine? Is this psychosocially balanced, and not a risk for insanity, worse where there are intentions of vice, to inflict pain? In comparison, the real jail is a correctional program on the whole, with rehabilitation and social activities to some extent for the well-behaved and lighter sentences.
5. In a very specialized area, with a sole talent/doctor manning the project, what happens to the clinics for severe and chronic cases like Cancer? Is there compensation for these patients – or they are to perish like 'lepers in quarantine'?
6. When there are situations which require litigation, especially, with regard to corrupt COVID officers, how can the isolated go about reporting?
7. Is there compensation for the dependence of 'the enclosed one' during the quarantine extension – we didn't find anything during the 3+weeks already gone? Shall we give a commutation of how our needs during the isolation have been met and obtain a refund?
8. Is there any radius permissible to walk in this extension as an allowance, in comparison to the first period?
9. Financial support – is it availed in compensation during the 'not-working' period?
10. Where the '*isolatee*' has other developing ailments, what is the time, travel, and freedom-to-see some private practitioner like, and where the isolation exacerbates some conditions and suffering, what shall be the considerations?

For the isolated is 'locked-in', and evil intents of the relevant 'securi-med' may be perpetrated without any observation by the victim or even the authorities. Danger lurks in such a program – when manned by those who have hearts burned with a burning hot-iron rod!

Progress report on *Wellness with regard to recuperation following the Malaria menace*

23-5-2020

- On this day I've prepared my first full supper dish of our traditional menu (since I returned from hospital)
- All along I've been having no reserve in the liver, despite double portions, so much more than my usual amounts. Yesterday and today, I've reverted naturally to my usual amounts of food in the plate – the liver's storage is getting more and more adequate. On the day of the journey to the private lab(3 days ago), I carried no victuals – only water
- No giddiness at all; and I feel like hoeing and digging in the garden soon
- My heart has some mild irregularity, but it gets better everyday
- Less fear of cold; as I type now, I have a waist-coat only, and not the jersey and the overcoat
- Less sleeping or resting episodes in the afternoon
- Phone attention is almost normal now
- Now, water is better tasting and loved again as the best drink in the world
- My voice is normal in pitch and volume and I can talk and sing well with clarity of lyrics again – those whom I speak with on the phone commend my vocal improvement back to its original

I hope I have at least cheered you my dear Reader; for when one reads a story, he may sympathize with a sufferer or some splendid character receiving injustice. It then so happens without noticing that this may affect the mind with strain or even stress. And now in my case, I write a true story of recent events in a setting of global corruption with wings and tentacles that may reach anyone, as humans are now so exposed and vulnerable!

So may my recovery above cheer thee and help in giving you the break before we cross over; yet remember to meditate well – for: The sins of actors to this day – **remain lurking** – and the searchlight of God needs to bring it into the open – expose for all to see – and enable blocking of evil strategies!

You might want to rest a while before we flip over unto: *Mutilation*!

CHAPTER SIX

MUTILATION

'Security' first in fists – Health last if not lost

It's now 0339hrs on 24/5/2020 as I type on my computer now. Last night, before I lay down to sleep, for some hours of recovery of my brain-drives, I spotted an article on the Italian doctors having 'discovered' that the microbiological 'perpetrator', causal agent, in 'COVID 19' SYNDROME-pattern is not viral, but **bacterial** – remember I have a shelf, and I have put this 'raw avocado' on the uppermost level – keen to see what shall become of it soon: Rottenness & fruit-flies? Or sound ripening and readiness for business in the Gastro-enteric Enterprise?

Whether true or not, there flashed something onto my mind:
The swab that gave me sinusitis!
If there was a pre-planned strategy to cause me harm, inoculation with bacteria would be easiest – and now the Italians are now claiming (following post-mortems they did against the WHO's cover-up inhibition of them) a bacterial causative agent!
And why does this retired soldier of an officer with the greatest zeal to persecute me to the end, insist, that some people have ended up testing positive after six weeks – does he know what they inoculated me with – and are aware it would make the test positive – as by way of the test, they have direct access to the nasopharyngeal site when they take the next swab – are they in waiting of the result of their 'business'? When you

deal with cadres of venomous guile and vile who have been granted so much power over your body, you cannot help thinking! The fact stands: They mutilated me in my sinuses – whether incidentally/accidentally or deliberately/intentionally? Who will prove?

I remember a conversation with a doctor, thinking I was talking to a fellow-colleague, and was trying to instil sanity into his senses for sound comprehension, and I said:

'Doctor, unless you are or you've been a soldier (with a past to regret over unjustifiable self-perpetrated horrible atrocities) or.......then I wouldn't have trouble why you wouldn't care the injustices you have perpetrated to this sufferer'

And the voice at the other end answered:

'In actual fact – I am indeed a soldier – I am a retired soldier – a retired colonel'

My own last:

'You have finished – don't go on!'

And I knew I only had to be careful for my life or for the life of my own, guard against this figure's intents – with prayers and supplications – not only of my own – but invited my prayerful fathers and brethren and family (Daniel 2v17-18)

When programs of this COVID nature come to Africa, **security** which is supposed to be for both victims and those to be protected from contraction of disease – risks 'contamination' with great abuse! From lurking hate, there can result horrible **mutilation** with debility and deaths which may even be passed as due to the threatening condition on the 'current market', yet evil-driven killers will murder as per their wish, if candidates for the security program are not selected carefully! Africa!

Also, do not be surprised when I say 'current market' – for the murderers high up on the NORTH and in the WEST, right now may be busy itching to be the first in the devil-driven competition, to make vaccines for testing, again where-else, but in Africa – on the sleeping black mothers and their babies, as the fathers are drugged from strange substances as in beer (not even the beer itself poisoning them) or in condoms etc. These Northerners

45

and Westerners and Easterners commit murders of continental and global degrees in silent and hidden genocides – unfortunately false Christendom, so much full in Africa's colonial influenced multi-sect worshiping, seems to make it even harder for the inner eye to be opened in order to see the dangers! Hence dangerous 'doctors' are elected in programs, who care only for the gold they are going to pan at the end of the day!

Here it might be the apt place to tell you about these gold panners, who mutilate without care for the future of seed currently in loins who shall come to the earth's surface tomorrow:

1. They effectively exert all their sun-drained labor – **for ultimate gains by corruptly licensed international mafias** in the West, North and East
2. They are **so mutilating** such as to kill themselves or even their own, including their kin – they don't just destroy rivers and other environmental havens
3. They have **no rules** and everything goes and nothing can really stop them from doing harm especially if corruption is rife in national and international markets and programs
4. They **do whatsoever allows them to earn a short-term living** – no care of a structure or anyone
5. They **don't care if what they do affects others** in complications, even their own – even a thought of the consequences of jail, as in leaving their offspring without parental care, is quenched as by just a single pull of 'weed', as a puff of smoke and associated whiff of the dagga's scent is blown to disappear, as they will soon disappear without realizing it – whilst holding the few notes of 'uneven sharing'
6. Where gold panning is rife (with its indication of allowable highest degrees of corruption – 'permissible' of crimes up to murder), **economies shrink**
7. They **know not a sorry**, neither remorse nor kindness – an expression of it being almost always derision
8. They are **ready to kill**, any time, and with immediate hiding of evidence

9. Given an opportunity, they can be easily **in league with the most evil of foreigners** – even with deals to the extent of human trafficking if not organ-trafficking (remember the slave-trade – many think it was over?!)

10. They ever **live in poverty** after mining the greatest of mineral strength – ending up with the terrible catastrophes too including the downloaded HIV

Why do you think I have elucidated the above - about gold-panners?

Because the team who injured me – I have seen them to be exactly like that! Mutilators! COVID-corruption masters! Money mongers! 'I-Don't-Carers'!

And if they wanted to kill me, what could have stopped them, as long as I would in pitiful fear, be at their disposal to access my body at their will?

I cannot close this topic before I tell thee how God has made me progressively conquer what I have so labelled the **Sinister Sinusitis**, perpetrated by those I thought were colleagues – the villagers would just have been glad to shower them the 'glory' of 'doctors'! Doctors? No – not for the moment – unless if in life they are someday converted to do no harm – and should they do it by mistake acknowledge and take responsibility!

The victory over Sinister Sinusitis

It was on day 2 (post swab-test) that I noticed Para-nasal Sinus irritation. I trust had I been in my original fitness before the Malaria infestation, my defense could have resisted whatever it was, except may be deliberate inoculation. I have a tendency to make diagnoses in the earliest stages of disease without so much missing – and on this second day post-swabbing, I felt all four on the right: the Maxillary, Sphenoidal, Frontal, and the Ethmoidal sinuses as inflamed. The irritation was still a bit low but it was a real bother, more-so with the anxiety and pressure of: 'What could they have done unto me?'

My lack of trust of the duo had quite a sound and indisputable basis. (Recall the unfair break in the middle of my anti-Malarial treatment for two days, whilst enclosed in the ward!) Steadily the pain increased each day, and I think on the third I was 100% sure I was afflicted in my sinuses. I started fomentations – breathing water-vapor from boiled 'gumtree'/ Eucalyptus leaves – in about 5litres of water boiled over 15-30minutes. The relief was great, doing the exercise 3 times a day. The teeth sensitivity on the entire right side would temporarily cease – it was exacerbated by cold, and keeping warm with direct compression of the right side with a hot water bottle was exceptionally helpful, though relief didn't last long. Headaches would become better for a little bit longer, but they would wake me as soon as the temperatures would fall in the twilight hours. That associated sensitivity of right sided teeth was constantly troublesome at night, with sleep-disturbing soreness!

Then I would take oral herbs of prescription class from our NFH list – a particular formulation has been so helpful to this day, apparently more than antibiotics. For my colleague, fearing the consequences of abscess formation in the special cavities, or Chronic Sinusitis, had persuaded me not to refute the course of Augmentin/Metronidazole that he prescribed.

I must say, I haven't been an antibiotic person; neither do I tolerate pills, nor do I remember having taken any pharmaceutical medicine over the past 10years. My body has indeed felt the strain from handling the injectable anti-Malarials, the subsequent orals, and finally the antibiotics with the painkillers – the latter that I am a full two days without touching now, having taken them sparingly. I hope in two to three days' time, I do finish my courses. It is my wish that God helps in the keeping of my soul's 'temple' as has been over these past ten years.

I have lived a 99%+ natural life-style – my acquaintances can testify – and I have known that those who don't take sugar or sugar-added foods don't succumb to Malaria – their body's in-built defense remains soundly intact and clears it for them. I wondered, when I first felt the Malaria-symptoms about 6 weeks before I was carried to the hospital – for I hardly need a test to diagnose Malaria, only to confirm it. I realized later as I self-reviewed my history, that prior to the period that I went near Mozambique border, about two weeks before the attack, I had been abusing oranges from our own trees – and indeed their sugar may be just as the commercial sugar in lowering defense, if abused. This is what corrupted my body, compromised me to fall into to the rugged-potholes, of the money-hungry **Corruption Of Virology** that **Instigates Dehumanization** Gold-panning program, running from the NORTH all the way down to the SOUTH. And upon the incidental positive test, I suffered the first-mutilation physically and psychologically from the cruel-neglect that denied me that rightful antimalarial treatment for two days.

Writing has discharged a lot of my strain and stress from this Captivity of a complex corrupt-maze. I wonder what added consequences will be suffered under the mask, glove and disinfectant program which is the other money-mongering line!

The damage is done not to individuals alone but to belts of communities, with even greater potential for hidden sequel.

Wonder if we are not in the near future, going to end up with multiple cases of psychic disturbance? And soon the already early-started Winter-season is going to be at its peak – wonder how many false positives might come with the surge of flus and common-colds. It would also depend on the integrity of the tests, the cadres and the system all together – but it's all to do with borrowed 'knives' – and complaining of bluntness will sound stupid to the lender or donator or provider's ear.

Now to tail off this chapter, the admission was voluntary, but the discharge was imposed, so is the isolation and related mutilation. As they have been monitoring, let us see how they have translated and interpreted my recovery – Chapter 7 shall reveal. And let's compare how they are doing it in Europe.

CHAPTER SEVEN

---◎---

TRANSLATION & INTERPRETATION

'Recovering from COVID'

Someone, a migrant, phoned me, about 13/14 years back, from the UK, I think a lady, no longer quite sure which one – these were her words:

'Now that you have (as a nation) *allowed the 'Easteners' to enter our territory, you are going to have **flus** in every season'*

I put this on one of the shelves of my mind's 'libraries'. Not two years were to pass before 'white moths' emerged from 'brown pupae'. It was true. The flu attacks in every month and every season confirmed her statement. I don't understand how she had got to understand about the 'Easterners' and flus, but I don't believe she had been to famous Eastern World herself at any stage in her life.

Flu was no more a Winter-disease, and the Winter-peak would be difficult to observe, because the disease became rife – finding it anytime and any day!

Within five if not slightly more years, I remember some vaccination exercise passed by, especially because the after-effects of the vaccine nearly killed some close one of us. Soon news about H1N1 would be a regular in our newspapers. I remember acquaintances asking me so much about H1N1 in those days, and I trust I had something to tell them sensible as a doctor who has since been wary to be equipped with information.

But how would I have guessed that some planned business was 'cooking' in the laboratories that early, for the future self-interests of a few. And in this day, information not disputable, flows with facts that there was indeed vaccination in early 2019 against 'flu', scientifically alleged H1N1, in the most troubled European nation of Italy.

The East remains secretive and not so readable, like their 'Hieroglyphics', oh no, sorry, MMMMM! While the West in official media demonstrates in bellows of blaming the East's laboratories - which sound scientist has not read the news, even between the lines that, as a matter of fact, corrupt scientific administrators of the West collaborated with the East, in the 'synthesis' of this evil pathogen?

And my question remains to this day: 'Why has God allowed it to spill in their nations first before the Southern hemisphere, where it would satisfy so much, the hearts of those who brewed the Human Immuno-deficiency Virus (HIV)?

And what is it about Italy that keeps this European nation in the 'limelight', for didn't a scientific guru from France discover, and wrote a paper about the truth of this Acquired ImmunoDeficiency Syndrome, as the Italian nation did present some patients troubled with the HIV disease then? Is not therefore the entire scientific community surprised about the position of Italy again in COVID-19?

But I have preferred the earnest searching of the Italian doctors and their consistent endeavor to define the disease to be clear from its syndrome pattern up to autopsy findings. They have been the first to breach officially that questionable forbiddance by the WHO COVID rules not to do autopsy.

And it is here I come, the Italian doctors and quite a number of American doctors, wonder, why they are being enticed or encouraged to put the CAUSALITY of death as COVID, where an obvious co-existing disease (with a positive COVID-test and not COVID-disease) is an obvious cause of death. An attractive payment for such a written death-certificate, to the doctor who 'abides', is reported to attract thousands for the transaction into his bank accounts – COVID CORRUPTION!

Now if this is happening, in the revered scientific world, what will the doctors in Africa make of COVID in diagnosis – how do they translate the findings, clinically and investigatory-wise – to come up with the conclusion that the suffering is due to COVID 19?

Let's come back to our 'arena'

I was admitted at the height of Malaria, with a 20% parasitemia found in my blood. Had I died before Day 4, I trust the cause of death on the certificate would have read: **MALARIA.**

Take the other side now, if I would happen to die after Day 4, the pattern of translation I have seen, would have put the number one cause of death as: *COVID-19!* Poor!

The corruption started in the West, North and East (WNE), and downloaded southerly, it doesn't lose its 'venomous' guile. Taking a look at a chart posted by the COVID team, a friend could read after my second swabbing (post-admission) was negative, that I was labelled as a case *recovered* from COVID-19?! It was my hope to be able to post that chart, but somehow it has gone out of my reach. I have kept the space, lest I find it!

TABLE send by Pastor that morning of that private lab result:

Where are our capable minds? Doesn't this 'security' program have some true medical consultants of a sound mind within it?

I **never** had COVID disease, before my admission, at admission (when the first swab-sample was taken), during admission, and after admission – unto this day, at least four weeks post admission.

Besides, all my two colleagues who treated me, and all the ward staff, all our team of ten workers including their families for those with family, plus my own household, Pastor and his own household, have all proven negative on that hailed 'PCR' test. And they were all followed up, and none was found during the 14days of quarantine, to have a temperature or any symptoms considered to be of COVID, even of any other disease. After all, myself, I never had any ongoing temperature, or relapse of fever, after it significantly came down on the second day of anti-Malarial injections. Had the positive COVID-test result been availed at the time of admission (if it were possible), out of scientific principle I would have suggested a second test immediately after the temperature had come down. But I wonder what would happen in the event of an immediate COVID-test result, for the security team and its proven brutality would have taken over – and the diagnosis they would entertain is COVID, not MALARIA; for they even couldn't continue my treatment of Malaria when it was necessary, rather enclosing me for two days with nothing, as my doctors I guess were already in self-quarantine.

Wonder where the evil kick would have landed me, had there been a quick/rapid result!

How about the local officer in charge of health – his own translation?

This one's questions demonstrate a lot of naïve traits, even if he himself might probably be not that naïve, but full of guilt. He phoned me about three times, to find out if I was not developing any 'flu-like symptoms', or cough or febrile feelings – he seemed to expect the positive COVID test to be soon matched. Surprisingly he never came to see me, for an assessment in the 'sea-diver's suit, to prove that I really didn't have these. I wonder if he would have any idea of what else to look for or expect in a patient supposed to have real COVID disease. But those three above, I suppose he could have been taught by some equally naïve 'company' from the big-city's security program, to enquire on just that 'triad'! All his subsequent phone calls were a bother. When you come to the Epilogue, I trust I shall be having enough data to prove to you dear Reader, why this local officer's phone calls were a bother. The counterpart duo on their visit, somehow, would make enquiry on whether he had ever come to see me, to which a 'nope' was always the answer – wonder why they would ask?!

Family and work-team

My son James trusts me. And he knows how I so much love him, that had I had the conviction or convincement that I had COVID disease, I would never have allowed him to see me. So does Mum – the mother who still bears within her, that womb that carried me for 9+months.

I have thanked God, that my beloved son Frank, has not gone otherwise, but accepted me as I presented myself. The attitudes of Tinotenda and Newton too were so much excellent, though reservations may still have to be left to God about a person's heart. Otherwise I saw no action in a single one of them that segregated me in the least. The Big City team of our shop – Zeph, Ane and Inno – literally would carry me on their laps – indeed never segregated me. They were with me up to the end. I must say, Inno suffered a terrible form of segregation in the location where he stays, but it was a 'worthy' and wealthy experience for a strong-hearted young-man. He shall emerge even stronger after it all. It is my hope, that towards the final pages, you shall read a brief account of his testimony on his encounters with COVID corruption, should he be willing! Young Nomore requested to visit, all the way from our project-site based towards Mozambique border. He was not afraid and showed no 'inch' of segregation in his mind. He brought me a bucket of shelled nuts to make peanut butter, plus 7.5litres of cows' milk (organic). Takudzwa, I haven't seen yet post-admission, but his voice has ever been sweet and his affection I have ever felt on the phone. Our old granny in the garden project had been coming to work, but she had to be stopped by a team on the lower ranks of the 'security' program – I wonder how much they gained in reaching her long distance homestead daily in terms of claims and allowances. You would think these travelers had been converted by a COVID 'goddess' into dedicated health workers! Ah! Since when? Dirty moneys!

Only one of our workers kept his distance on his own – drawing to the garden only to take his money for the month – disappeared without telling us a word until his COVID daily-assessors' visits dried too. That one, he showed signs of fear of contracting disease, I really think so. I made sure, I sent him to work in a faraway post of our work where he would return for a week to his family after every three weeks. At least he would be safer there, away from my presence till 'I don't know' - when the 'COVID-contagion' would be well decayed in me for sure!

Overall, I thank all our team and my family for trusting God. They have also believed and learnt avidly, the lessons I have taught them over the years.

When COVID comes as in the West, North & East (WNE)

Should COVID-19 appear on our arena, as it is in the WNE, not only the translation and interpretation will change – but the workers will change – money mongers are likely to go into hiding – only a few dedicated workers will remain as front-line. How many of the latter does Africa have? A concerned Swiss lady, has said unto me: 'I wish this disease doesn't come to Africa!'

The positive test has arrived, and that: 'full time!', as Zimbabwean young generation would love to express on their corrupted tongues, but the disease, indeed COVID disease, is yet to arrive 'big time'!

Dear Reader, mark my words.

Doesn't Chapter 8 say?!:-

Wait until the Real COVID arrives!

CHAPTER EIGHT

◌

SURVEILLANCE

'Wait until the Real COVID arrives!'

Take a picture! I'll take mine! Of a doctor – a father of five children, the eldest in University, the smallest one on the mother's laps, all the middle ones in school – the second in late high school, the middle one in late primary class and the remaining one in preschool. That would sound like computerized 'ideal' spacing! Yet that's not the point.

This is in Southern Africa, and COVID-19 **disease** has showed its arrival without need of tests, and no need to hear from an enemy's unethical & illegal report, even a medical colleague igniting the whatsapp, that Dr Wisdom C GWATIDZO has tested positive for COVID, yet the latter doesn't even suffer the disease. But the disease now talks on its own, far-away from the laboratories, both state-run and private ones, the latter having made real 'kills' on companies, currently 'safely' screening asymptomatic workers for 65 United States Dollars per person!

Will this father, if he is a dedicated one, go for work excited? Picture his goodbye to his dear ones. Picture him in those garments with the very sick, the ones in the Intensive Care Unit (ICU), and the dead bodies – for he has to certify deaths, and this time really script it truly COVID-19, not imaginary, borderline or far-fetched, but indeed realistic. And doctors in our locality, now have the chance to learn what the WNE doctors have had to go through; yet how many will survive to tell the stories to their families, to put them in journals, to write books and papers?

I better finish mine soonest! But I trust God shall preserve me to his own hour.

Below I give you a glimpse through a pinhole - the relevant stations of my predicted observations:

1. Clinics
2. Hospitals
3. Police posts and stations and camps and roadblocks
4. Soldiers - where-so-ever they may be
5. High density townships
6. Low density suburbs
7. The villages

Let's get moving – this is Africa! The dramas and drills are over. The real time has come: And in a fictitious approach, an old retired doctor-friend, has sent me views from over in their land of the North-Eastern zone – and I have written it mostly like my own story!

Clinics

Pregnant mothers there? For ANC? That's a lie! What of for delivery? Don't you know that the 'Mbuya Nyamukutas', those traditional midwives are back in the villages and towns, and they are training their own subordinates and helpers due to demand? Why? Isn't the lockdown emphasizing safe-distancing in the bedrooms? Babies are still coming! Yet they say we are going to be with COVID for some time, and some rules might seem to be as though forever?!

Where's the nurse, yes, the Sister?

Some people are waiting with a scotch-cart? Donkey pulled? Yes? But where is the nurse? The doors are closed.

Find yourself answers – pray that it doesn't come to Africa.

And beware – **certain fiction-like material has sometimes come to pass** – here it goes! Now we know of long-back films that talked about a deadly Corona Virus! Coincidence?

Hospitals

Hospitals? There's even a story. They got some sort of preparedness when Dr Wisdom C GWATIDZO's counterpart, a Dr Yamiko KAMUTU in the Northern country got a positive COVID test as Case No. 23 of Mutsinje village in MATANDWE (wonder why subsequent cases were not to be labelled by destination)

But there is this particular hospital, so pathetic, somewhere in the East. The local hospital's Admin-doctor there is said to have suffered many complications of multiple diseases. The action group had so much respect for him due to his role during the drill-era, for his contributions especially around the case of Mutsinje Village, Matandwe, were tremendous. They then chose only to put on his death certificate, Diabetes Mellitus and Hypertension. However the villagers have been known to have rumored that AIDS must have been the number two cause. They were hinting at COVID having ripened all the other illnesses into an inflammatory tumorous state of most organs in his body. His burial – no one knows – we could have asked his friends, but they are since gone. How about the hospital where he worked?

The maternity ward is closed. They say the trained midwives claimed an excessive COVID allowance and were denied. In-patients is closed. The mortuary man, a 'Yao'-descendant is said to be the busiest, but since administration is shaky, he's worried about the electric maintenance of the 'fridges' or 'cold rooms' as he calls them with a tinge of the vernacular 'accent' . The technician cannot be found. An ambulance is said once to have been sent to his home further Easterly, but it was gossiped he had hidden in a cave of a huge mountain, where resides '*Nyamubobo*' – the **'Flying Snake'** (*Mubobo* in Chewa) – unfortunately he never came back. Now in superstitious Africa, it becomes difficult to decipher what's real.

It's a reminder to me of the famous story of Makate and his people in Mutoko.

It has been said that the mortuary man is now amongst the highest on the COVID-bribery list which comes out in the newspaper weekly. The richest business man in the district and another one who works at the courts have been rumored to have vowed to intend to revive the hospital services fully – though their intent to convert a number of wards into 'cold-rooms' has been an evening debate in the round-huts of villagers whose homesteads are lucky to have 'numbers'. 'It is still a wonder how these two men are still surviving', the villagers say and applaud, but no more with the single clap & clatter against one another's hand – for the former resident doctor had warned them sternly during the drill-era when only one case was positive (yet not COVID-diseased!).

You can finish for yourself with regards to the rest around the hospital – the rowdy grassy grounds, cut-down Jacaranda trees by neighboring villagers for the cold winter, squirrels no more in the ceilings only, but making a zoo for the cheapest tourist through the windows, and where there's a rat, there's a cat! Yes! COVID arrived! Did the first 'front-liners' get a chance to 'eat' their money? If not, how about those who inherited those corrupt 'COVID-riches' – will they live to eat those moneys?

Police camps, stations & posts & roadblocks

The drill era is past!

One passer-by observes: there is an argument. One 'boss' has fallen with another 'chef', who has sent his still lower-rank son to the road-block along the highway that leads to a Northern country. He even shouts:

'Go get my son now! If he's to die – you'll pay for it beyond all the junky-earnings you've made from COVID!'

The arrival of a bigger van with a huge and taller fellow of 'engulfing' superior rank, sees the two follow into a 'hotel'-like office that a smart junior rushes to unlock and open the door thereof – the eye-witness proceeds with his journey to seek if any shop is open for purchasing at least a small tablet of soap. In the past soldiers used to 'man' the shopping centres! Now, where are warehouses still full of items to continue supplying these retail shops in Africa, having 'sold' if not slain Industry, to rely on 'Eastern imports'? He shall try anyway, and so, he meets me along the most recent tarmac and gives me the story!

Roadblocks were popular during the Drama era. But the few survivors among the temporary traffic support staff, 'see no more need of them'! See no more need of them? What we have learnt, vehicles after some brief surge, when the real disease started 'digging and menacing', have become too few to earn a traffic officer some 'COVID dollars', unless a sympathizer litters a few dirty local currency onto the ground as if by error – the officer after-all is no longer 'fierce' or 'fearsome'. Yet still another factor – new-looking vehicles that now traverse the provinces along trunk-routes are either the 'COVID vehicles', some with 'whitish' faces, now said to be among the team to 'help'! (Window panels have a deep tint, but it has been rumored it could be Eastern 'friends' of the nation?!)

If I am to go on, my story would be too long, but get a relation who is still in the police if your family still has a survivor, he can tell you what's on the ground?

But before I close this 'police section', have I told you that police posts, which had now been turned into COVID-satellite cabins have been closed – 'numbers' are no longer enough to man them.

Also, the overlap of the time-period between drill cases and real cases was hideous; and it is suspected, since everyone then had desired to go and siphon COVID-bribes – most must have contracted as they dealt with 'informal funeral' vehicle drivers and mourners, without realizing that the flood-gates had been untimely opened upstream of the river they 'lavished' to swim in. Today, police in block-attendance, not by will of course, but by reason of duty as per their pledge - they hardly stop vehicles! Masks are no longer the rule, wonder how that changed; maybe new observations in the WNE scientific community. Phones are said to be 5G and handsets and airtime are unaffordable for most. So the officer at the block has not much link with the station, as most roadblocks are set on non-built middle-of-bush stops, with bush toilets for both the officers and the travelers – Oh! COVID Hygiene?!

Where are the military officers that used to help them on the highway?

Soldiers - where-so-ever they may be

The parliament is rumored to have only 30 original members left. The contraction of COVID disease of these 'biggers' has been more of hushed, and some who have been thought to be sick at home, are suspects of death without hero-ship status. Who would take them to the heroes anyway, and what crowd, in the social distancing era? Capable drivers of the special limousine-hearses are also said to be in hiding in their villages, and the private funeral services seem to have parked a large number of their fleets due to loss of drivers – so they are now too expensive.

New helpers in parliament seem not announced yet.

But it has been said there's now a cure. Brought from where? Of course, from the East? But they need a deal brokered! And there has been a division and disagreement amongst the heads of the nations.

Soldiers have already been 'vaccinated' by marshal law. And they are up in the villages and townships to ensure that everyone is 'vaccinated'.

One leader is aware of hazards of inoculation that may wipe away populations, but the other, even if he would be aware, or even not, 'A rule is a rule; it's got to be followed; we just need the country to get going especially when *friends* offer help – marshal law is for the Army and the Masses together – they fight alongside one another!'

Soldiers are busy campaigning for vaccination in suburbs and villages with their guns and bandoleers visible to scare in open daylight. They used to be in the townships during the COVID-drama era, but businesses have since closed and there are no more people there.

How shall be the vaccination, of everyone in accordance to a so called GB, in order to bring the world again to normalcy? Yah? One would wonder: Is our Africa going to survive? May be the slave-trade era was better? What kind of suffering can be envisaged in this sad era about to fall on the people?

'Aren't the soldiers African to think African?'

Some two strangely remaining white bearded and bold-headed 'centurion' old men were chatting!

The other, seemingly of scholarly descent in appearance, with his tier on, and a suit plus a cloak on top to cover him for the breeze, would answer: 'Soldiers in most nations, I have gathered, live from their early training days, on a special diet and 'drugs' allowable to them, to ensure a particular mindset – leading them to think more patriotic as to win a battle, but not necessarily to consider their populations' wellness security. But to qualify it better, these inputs that alter their attitude to humanity, are not from African countries or governments – but from the 'Biggies' of the West, North or East that they may be more in *league, in link, in ally or in friendship* with!'

'So that is why you were not keen to send your son – I hope they are not going to beat the people into the vaccination when it starts!' the shorter one echoed in rhetoric. And they parted and disappeared. A young son told Adala Chilombo his father this one – he had been in a Sycamore tree in these days of spontaneous meal-rationing, to eat a few figs the birds had been 'kind' to pierce but not finish, when he overheard the two – his mind is magnetic and his memory telegraphic!

High density suburbs

Zimbabweans like to say '**Chabvondoka**', especially the young generation, the term a local officer used when only one person who was not even sick of COVID incidentally tested positive for it. It actually means: **the tribulation has actually or really started now!**

Those who had died would be said of them by the living: '*Vakafa havana chavakavona*', meaning '**The dead must never have seen or experienced anything like such during their lifetime!'**

In town they are aware, some go inside and lock their doors, only to unlock them due to tear gas – they have to line-up for a **vaccine-with-a-signature** – the Mr. GB from the West needs all New World order global citizens to be clean!

Those already on the queue, whisper, or cry or murmur or even grunt or whimper: '*Udzazikanira yani wee?*' and in our local vernacular: '*Unozvirambira aniko?*' meaning: 'To whose authority will you be able to refute it?

Two weeks are over, and there's hardly anyone stopped for examination by security, who doesn't have the mark!

Most of them wished they were residing in the low-density suburbs – where mostly chefs and their relations only, now live, in 'dura-walls' and guarded 'mono-lopolis' (cf. megalopolis)

But do they really know what's happening on the Easterly low-density suburb section?

Let's go down below.

Low density suburbs

The duration for the vaccination period lapsed in this area of elites. Mama Temba had been first with her sons after being encouraged by her white boss to be early. Other general hands and helpers who were living mostly in the so-called servants' quarters behind the main house followed suit. There was a rumor that their children would be checked at school, and any of them without the 'signature' would lead to a surveillance of their entire family at a severe penalty – and a 'catch', no vaccination would be effected without the parents of the child/student. Some single mothers had a terrible time to explain or to search for fathers they had never communicated with for years. But somehow in the end it was done.

Where were the elite, the owners of the properties, or if not, some nobles of foreign or local origin renting in them? They would be checked in blocks set by 'securics' around shopping malls, about filling stations and highways and tollgates – should they be found wanting, they were vaccinated at a penalty fee that 'cost a leg' – after-all they are the travelers; a number of them would be overheard on their phones by the helpers in their homes and the word of the common circulation was:

Down South, there is a safer vaccine and a lot were obtaining passes from Immigration at a biting cost, to pay again for the vaccine upon arrival in 'Gondwana-land' as if for a small car – it was all so prohibitory – but the fee covered an entire family and the elite loaded themselves and accomplished the journeys. This was where the Phase One COVID money, earned from the drills of punishing poor unfortunate guinea-pigs was squandered against their will. And tollgate fees where raised for those on such trips, tickets to be demanded for verification at the border post's local side before the cross-over. Should they be found to have cheated, there was again a penalty to slap their faces.

And it was rumored these were the ones 'going to live!' But others insisted in softest of whispers: 'We shall all die anyway.'

Yet, if a genocide was well planned to exit blacks out of Africa, those who received the free signature would perish in a marked period like all at once! No matter what reproduction would be done by the remainder, the rate would never multiply in time enough for safety in numbers. HIV/ AIDS already accomplished its part. The youngsters and children and remaining children have to go – can you read Mr. GB's mind?

And the remainder would not find time for being proud to anyone either. How would pride earn enjoyment with no subordinate or anyone lower to 'shine' at or to entice? The helpers would be gone too; and robots as of Rwanda would they be switched over to the job? Wonder which 'ally' gave Rwanda those donations in the COVID-Drill-era? Not really donations, but usually in exchange for raw minerals or materials of unimaginable value, should the processing be accomplished in the 'industrial country'. COVID corruption influence came to stay, with the almost permanent destruction of equilibrium.

With 5G, lessons were express on line with no glitches or delays – the unjustifiably despised 'lazy' and strained-down teachers had gone.

Only if these 'white'-blacks had known, that poor performers among them would soonest be like the Aborigines and Red-Indians. A few really capable talents would be kept till the master had copied thoroughly, this time without need of patenting, and till the 'slave' was drained thoroughly and comforted in dosing with planned beer, drinks, drugs and medicines stronger than evils of today.

The Villages

The chief voters of the powers of Africa, the masses, most of them living in abject poverty – where the genocidal 'engineer' Mr. GB sees them as useless inhabitants, better to be permanently removed to give space to 5G and development.

They would wake up early morning. The soldiers here had a hard time. Households dwell greatly more sparsely than in town. Roads have never been built for touristic travel, so access at night when they are back in the homesteads is a challenge – rivers have no fords – certain mountains which they have mastered to climb over years require a helicopter or a specialist mountain climber with his 'tools'.

They seemed to win at first, but the period had to be extended to 6months, so that each person would have the mark and the world would be clean – again to the means and end of Mr. GB and his team. Now an entire cluster or village would end up rounded by an adequate no. of security forces – and the three-pin punching began 'running'.

The effect of vaccination here would be stronger in apparent effect, dropping some lives 'there-n-there', but the master's plan had to be accomplished! Whether it would be because the subjects were tired from the escape of daylight on successive days, or possibly the dose was deliberately increased for the illiterate who cannot say much, who would know best except God!

The end of the simple and lovely though poor black man's village system was coming to an end.

Thank you Old man – Atate – Adala AChilombo for the glimpse from Upper North Easterly Territory?

Reader, instead of being angry, I hope you have been stimulated, and I trust you are going to alert others.

May you be relieved and comforted during the 'patience'-lesson below; we are back in the Garden Centre yet again.

CHAPTER NINE

— ☙ —

PATIENCE

'Have you been a patient patient?'

Someone in a faraway land, in one of the German-speaking nations, asked me the above question sometime during my recuperation, and I knew straightaway she meant: 'Have you been a patient with patience?'

The Christ would express it as **long suffering**.

And my Longman dictionary in agreement goes: the ability to **wait calmly** for a **long** time, and accept *delays* (I would add: + *inconveniences*) without becoming *angry* or *anxious*.

What a godly quality! Who needs it most? The Good Samaritan (in Luke Chapter Ten), possessed it, and he was patient with a patient. The patient seems to bear this name PATIENT, in order that the caregiver is reminded of the need to have patience with a patient.

A patient may not be themself. They may be strained or stressed in their mind by infirmity, especially over long periods of time, as with Aeneas (Acts 9v33). A patient may not be able to help themselves so much physically (like every able-bodied who may not realize their luck), and thus may need some very patient helper to bath them, dress them, feed them, help with exercise, and sometimes even help with the toilet.

At times the situation has been even more pathetic, requiring specialist bearers of love, loving-kindness and mercy knitted together in the patience-package; for sores, even as complex as gushes from deliberate injury, multiple pustules, or infected burns may change the air in the room and so the ventilation capacity is as though limited! Meanwhile diarrheas and melena-stool, rotting tumors and cancers, and dilapidating lungs may turn an entire ward into a *honey-sucker*'s leakage!

Yet on the other hand, severe splitting and throbbing headache as of a space occupying lesion, neural pain as of extensive Herpes Zoster and its connotations, pain of intestinal obstruction as of volvulus or intussusception – may be accompanied by groaning and tears (&mucus) and swearing if not together with cursing or a clear-cut shift from the sane-line!

Now, dear Reader, by the nomenclature – patient, who was meant more than the other to bear the other with patience, but the CAREGIVER who loves with patience – indeed the longsuffering, the forbearance, the love and loving-kindness?!
Only someone who doesn't seek an immediate reward can manage here – one who sees the rewards and benefits from their Lord in the distance to be reached someday.

I wouldn't argue with my 'superiors' who posed the question to me – about having been a patient patient – for I have never won any argument over them – they always tend to immediately win; only I suppose, when they in the long-run realize that they were actually on the wrong side, pitifully they cannot condescend to an inferior. The second chapter is full of my encounters whilst I was still a patient. To be enclosed for two days inside a ward with treatment that was supposed to continue, cruelly interrupted! And to be kicked out like a dog! Called out in names on the media, even as a 'colleague' would ignite it all! The type of patience for such a patient may only be derived from the example of Christ to one whose master is this Conqueror of the cross, who has invited his own to bear each one's cross. And I remember one lesson I never forget that our father – the great man of God gave us:

Why Christians Suffer?!

One quality that can heal a sufferer or even a persecuted one, is the spirit of forgiveness. It clears and cleans his/her mind. Such, don't brew a Cancer by brooding or breeding a mood! Instead they continue in doing good and eating real food and soul-bread, as they keep a sound mood with inner happiness that the Bible emphasizes - It helps them to heal:

Proverbs 17v22

A merry heart doeth good like a medicine:
But a broken spirit drieth the bones.

The immune system is loaded so much in the blood-producing bone-marrow, but the *'moody'*, finish their marrow to their peril, while the good boost it to their living. Where are you?

There is a type of Christianity that neglects accomplishing justice where it is called for. When God says do go ahead and bring certain issues and/or persons 'to the book', be persuaded enough to do it – it may help not only you but others today and 'tomorrow' – it might help to liberate or to change evil bills, rules and laws influenced by bad souls and evil spirits. But let it be truly God's will, and not your own will!

And the Wisdom of God doesn't justify quietness in matters which need talking in order to resolve issues (Matthew 18-20). Yet, this doesn't justify you to be angry with them, for this is the time you need to engage your heart wisely in order to win another's soul with words not rushed and never crushing, but calculated, well thought of and soundly judged (Proverbs 15v28, 16v23). And pray before you go, so that you are well-guarded against the unexpected evils and guiles and hypocrisy and haughtiness of the devil in the heart of the bringer of stumbling blocks.

I hardly reported cases of theft, especially if small items were involved, but even for bigger items. However I was pushed towards reporting one case, only to realize at the end of day that it was the Lord's act that led me to.

As soon as we entered with the robber, the charge office crammed with more people than for its room, suddenly had a commotion and noise of voices that changed the routine on the day – the police cadres taking statements dropped their pens! And some shouts would rise:

'What? That's my curtain!'

Another:

'My Iron!' with pointer finger towards the bucket.

Yet another offloading the pail:

'Ah! My radio!'

And it went on, till I questioned myself:

'Had the Lord not helped the villagers to run-after and catch him – how would all these people have retrieved their precious items?'

Just illustrative, when God says do it – go ahead and do it – as much as possible – and that without undue delay!

Anyway, everyone ought to be patient, both the patient and all who care for and mind them.

Let's go into the garden again

In the garden, into the garden, right into the corner of the garden, the very North-western Corner, into that Corner House, or fully named *St Andrew's Corner House* of memories, the very apartment where Atate on his trips to/fro Mozambique, loves to passby and lie his head for sleep – right into that precious and special little house all garden-inhabitants gather into for the early morning hour of **Bread** and **prayer**. Today 26-5-2020, we are going to examine closely, the way Jesus led a lawyer not only to the quality of practical longsuffering, but to the entire **Love** (see I John 4v8) that fuels it all with a demonstration of real patience by the Caregiver for the Patient:

Luke 10v25-37 begins where a proud lawyer was to 'eat **Bread**' and 'drink **Water**' without knowing it. And he would ask a question even of benefit to us all, 'Greeks' of this day. It must have been an equal surprise of Nicodemus' magnitude to him that Jesus knew his career, and gave address in a similar manner to the ignorant teacher and ruler of the Jews (who didn't know these things) – this lawyer received the first search-light question:

What is written in the law? How readest thou?

And on this occasion, the lawyer had to recite the written law-of-Love to its Author! The Author knew that the lawyer did not have the heavenly-package of such double LOVE upon his heart, but as the (best) Teacher – beyond the initial imagination by Nicodemus of a Rabbi – **The Lord** allowed him to start like a kindergarten child – recitation.

This law has two components. The **first** can be imitated so easily by a Priest, a Levite or a Congregant or Chorister in their colorful neat garment – to '*make-believe*' in the eyes of the passerby that they must be bearing the Love of God.

Yet this first law doesn't live alone on a real child of God, but it lives bound to the **second** law of **love thy neighbor** as thyself!

Thus the Love of The Father and The Son who have come to dwell in the heart of their beloved, can be there, silent like electricity in the pylons. But somewhere, at 'destinations', 'sites' or 'occasions' and 'occurrences', one can point to an action-site or centre-of-play:- here there are no short-cuts or else a short might cause fire or disaster! Hence, the second demonstrates the love in the arena where other inhabitants are walking, working and worshipping (or praying). Don't think yet, wait a little, about the man who has planned, with equally evil-minded friends to decimate the black and whatever populations they deem useless – he has his own 'church' where he was 'baptized' and regularly goes to!

Let us rather dwell on the same level as the lawyer in order to benefit from the Real Writer, so that He may engrave this dual-LOVE-law upon each one's heart.

And hear the Lord – '*answered right*', yes in the lesson – yet 'this **do**' on the practical-field test – the result = LIFE!

Eeeeeh! Amazing!

Double LOVE portion .... Spiritual life addition

A slow law student would have probably have questioned:

'You mean I hadn't started living?

But a hearkening law candidate would set a landmark – sinful past behind – and life of LOVE forwards ever!

And I would like to believe, our friend the lawyer was on the latter, thus beginning to be filled! With what? Wait until the **energizing-oil** comes, and the **healing-wine** too, altogether, for the soul's strength and for the body's wellness!

The first law, of course, would not trouble the lawyer, he could hide in his garment, his robes, his hood, his cap or even as in the pomp of King Agrippa and Bernice and be considered as very 'godly' – imagine how much King Agrippa would *answer* about The **W**ay, and even Paul would acknowledge, yet for the King **to walk** The Way was the desire of the Holy Ghost!

And true, the lawyer would not doubt about the first which had *short-term cover-up*, but, the second, which gave a question out of the challenges of **living with others** on the work- or playground, thus he would ask:

And who is my neighbor?

And here the lawyer earned us all a story! Of GLAD TIDINGS, indeed the GOSPEL! The Gospel of a good and true neighbor.

I have told you before that when COVID comes, then all the money-lovers will hide and disappear. And we ought to see those who operate with the love of God having taken their place.

Hopefully no one had considered the above a lie!

See the Priest pass, See the Levite leave, without touching the needy – even stripped (before garments get spoilt with blood & dirt – he must have been reverently dressed, otherwise why on earth would even a robber covet tatters) and eventually wounded and left for dead.

See the one who gave charge to the inn-keeper: 'Take care of him'; indeed a true Caregiver – the friend who comes **down** his high seat upon the high vehicle, to be at the same level as the sufferer – ensure the immediate first aid – ensuring he can lift and saddle him with less wail.

I presume such Caregiver, as his counterpart, also on a journey, but not feeling delayed when it comes to pouring of LOVE, wouldn't lack change-clothes in his rucksack or purse-string bag – and fail would he not, to spare them for the sufferer for fear of spoiling with blood!

See the Caregiver call at the inn-entry. Warding transactions not to be delayed, payments later – there is someone who earnestly needs a place to rest urgently! On the morrow, the healing must have showed, for the Caregiver wouldn't have rushed – indeed God's love heals. At a mission-station, where dwelleth brethren filled with the love of God – erring souls are healed and weary bodies are healed too, indeed made whole! The end result: The entire beast is made whole! A love that knows no expenses but even spending one's entire self for soul-winning! Even the extra two coins can be sacrificed without an outcry, for when the review is done, the wonderful Lord (who reassured: 'to take no thought' on what to eat, drink or wear - Matthew 6v33) will have provided for his own.

For this type is never a manner of love that wouldn't leave the sufferer untransformed, or even unconverted! Imagine the kind of wholesome meditation in the Lord that the lucky, delivered-one, engaged in his thoughts. I can picture him by or about the inn wondering like the blind one of John 9, on when he would meet and see his **Angel** again – to give thanksgiving and glorification.

Picture that **Angel**, the Lord, even the **Good Samaritan**, who never takes bribe or what is not his – Acts20v33. He harvests and earns from his own mission or work-fields to gather not only for himself alone, but for the lives of others as well – Acts 20v34.

And he imparts influence on the healed one to get fit for the mission-field, and so eventually laboring to think and plan and **do** for others, even to 'support the weak' and to remember that **W**ord from the Lord Jesus: '**It is more blessed to give than to receive.**' Acts 20v35

We found the occasion to humble ourselves in prayer in that old-fashioned corner-house! God is kind. Amen.

After prayer:

I had to thank the three who joined me in prayer – for accepting the Wisdom of God never to reject me; remember, I had been treated as a COVeeD by the smart ones.

Wait, you shall be quite fully enlightened after Chapter 10, plus reading the testimonies of a few who suffered the 'COVID'-travail together with me for the sake of Truth (II Timothy 2v3).

Now - Spiritual freedom can still come today, but how (?) about freedom from COVID CORRUPTION: –

See chapter 10.

CHAPTER TEN

—— ✺ ——

FREEDOM

For how long? – beware: Deadly vaccine!!

There are two types of **fear** as well-defined by the Lord Jesus – one is a **de**structive fear that denies one freedom – the other is the **con**structive fear that earns a soul real freedom while living in this life:

Who was Jesus addressing? – 'Friends'

Luke12v4
'Be **not** afraid of them that kill the body, and after that have no more that they can do' (Type I)

Luke12v5
'But I shall forewarn you whom ye shall fear: Fear HIM, which after HE hath killed hath power to cast into hell; yea, I say unto you, Fear HIM.' (Type II)

There the two fears stand-out clearly beyond doubt. One type must substitute the other, at some turning-point in his/her life. Type II fear casts out Type I fear, whereby True Freedom enters a person's life.

Hence listen to the confidence of the changed Paul – The Apostle (as opposed to the old Saul – 'Chiefest' of Sinners): (Hebrews 13v6)
'..........I will **not** fear what man shall do unto me'

And in demonstration of great growth in grace the Apostle reveals even more:

'Who shall separate us from the love of Christ?' (Romans 8v35)

And he challengingly goes:

- Shall tribulation
- Or distress
- Or persecution
- Or famine
- Or peril
- Or sword

Even fearlessly declaring:

'As it is written, For thy sake we are killed all the day long: we are accounted as sheep for the slaughter. (Romans 8v36)

Then in the 9th chapter of his epistle to the same Romans, the 29th verse, The Holy Ghost in Paul demonstrates **the risk of an entire Nation** from peril due to gross *lack* of the fear of God, as Paul quotes the Prophet Esaias:

'Except the Lord of Sabaoth had left us a seed, we had been as Sodoma, and been made like unto Gomorrha.'

The signs of peril of such nations having been spelled out clearly to Abraham by God himself (Genesis 18v20):

'.....Because the cry of Sodom and Gomorrah is great, and because their sin is very grievous;'

One would wonder, what a grievous type of sin conceived the COVID virus concept in the minds of the murderers and genocidal plotters, and what level of grievous sin would make God allow multinationals to perish from the corrupt COVID-peril!

'Days are evil!' (And hear the Apostle warn again)

Yet a person can earn freedom – by allowing his/her **soul** to be a 'true worshipper' of the Father 'in spirit and in truth' (John 4v23&24)

And nations are at least 'free' – when they allow souls to be preached the Truth to, in order that **the-whosoever-will** may truly worship God – The Spirit, 'in spirit and in truth' – as Christ and the Holy Ghost tell all things of the Kingdom of Real freedom (freedom from sinful-living).

Why the COVID experience?

It was flashed on my mind on the afternoon of the 29th of May 2020:
Why would God allow my poor self as a sheep in the middle of wolves, to experience the COVID persecution, even without the COVID disease?

And the answer was flashed immediately:
Because I wouldn't have seen the corruption as vividly as I did perceive it so thoroughly from inside the circle, encompassed by the persecuting corrupt COVID 'actors' in that corrupted action-cycle!

Had I not been exposed to the segregation and persecution which comes with COVID-discrimination, I doubt if this book would have come into existence. And I have the conviction that like 'everyone-else' – I would have been fooled to believe that most seemingly 'proven' cases (indeed potentially false-positive) of the 'drama-phase' are genuine positive cases! Thank God who was happy that I shouldn't remain in that ignorant position.

The decimation already done and threat of further decimation

The corruption of the WNE will always find its own roads & pathways, its own doors and access-holes, its own organ-systems plus its typical personnel – matching corrupt pathways to the result of killing deceptively, murdering silently, exterminating massively and decimating till there is no security in numbers!

The most painful part of it to a vigilant philanthropist and patriot, is the downloaded effect of the corruption from the superior world, in avidly drawing covetous and money hungry enslaving masters and killers from the very populations that are being decimated! And it doesn't matter the level of intellect, be it a trained nurse or more-so one with specialty like a midwife, a 'brilliant' (in knowledge of drugs & drug-lists) junior doctor or a consultant professor of renown (in tropical medicine or even pediatrics), not to mention social workers who are like hacked, and imitating lawyers who never dared to find values in the traditional laws and systems that preserved their nations in the past!

It is so painful!

And it makes the threat to our vulnerable populations more profound – worse should vaccination arrive!

The HIV-exterminating phase proved naivety and short-sightedness on the locals

In 1992, I was doing final year Bachelor of Medicine and Bachelor of Surgery. And during that period, Pediatricians were teaching us:

'Majority of children with HIV/AIDS, die in their first year or second year of life!'

We saw and witnessed the experience, as we were mostly practical on the wards – it was pathetic! Imagine the suffering of parents, as they lost their seed and heirs – oh the anguish and helplessness and stigma too! Imagine the commotion within the immediate and extended families! Separations by premature end of life in marriages if not divorce whereby a partner (especially the breadwinners or 'elite' class of women) would just abandon the family by seeking a livelihood in a far and distant area – hence some numerous migrations among the working class, even across borders and over the seas!

Yet the learned consultants would be blinded enough, possibly, through 'bait' moneys in the 'land-cruiser' programs, never to see the hidden inoculations coupled in the formalized yet deadly vaccines for the so-called 'immunizable' conditions – at that time they were sung from kindergarten and granted and 'confirmed' up to the medical and post-grad school as six immunizable conditions, and the '*The Road to Health*' CARD (weight/height growth assessment chart of a child) became like a 'passport' since then, for a child's entry into school.

So a parent, had naively, to ensure vaccination of the child, in order not to miss the opportunity of education of their offspring! What a trap!

It is at this stage that I have my greatest single appreciation of the so-called 'MAPOSTORI' (the white-robed 'Apostolic-sect' of old)!

Who doesn't know their escape history of vaccinations?!

And medical and pharmaceutical intelligence would view there dodging as 'stupid' and 'ignorant' and what-you-name-it?

Let Africa examine and review history again today, and re-judge the act of this sect with regard to immunization.

Let Consultants of Africa be humble enough to study well, the gains of this 'Apostolic-sect', in not vaccinating its offspring – especially by looking at those existing among them from the birth registry of 1992 +/- 1. Distortion of results may only emanate from ongoing hidden biological warfare, but at least something could be appreciated.

Am I trying to promote boycotting of immunizations? No! So long as it's not the biological extermination program. But how then can one distinguish, given that it is not something derived and administered from our own communities and populations, but an import, in this lethal era – of toxic agents!

Hence the brains of survivors are already 'cooked' by the stage of brain-maturation, so that the future of their minds and thinking, with regard to invention and practical valuable creativity is marred or 'perfectly' inhibited – hence Africa to remain the permanent slave!

Now robots and technology have necessitated the removal of the necessity of human-slavery – and 5G new world-order techniques prefer elimination of the 'useless' community from their God-given lands, in order for 'free' (yet in reality **bloody**) possession of the gold, the emeralds, the diamonds, the tantalite, the platinum and whatsoever Africa cannot industrially account for in ultra-extraction and utmost-purifications – let-alone the processing and manufacturing!

But like one eventually-blind politician of old in the so-called 'Area C' about Mudzi area, beyond Mutoko of Zimbabwe, said to the first colonialists in court:

'If a blind man is living in a beautiful and rich vast area, given him by God – would you take that land from him because he is blind?'

Of course I won't mention his name, after-all he's since gone to be with his ancestors, and I know it would make some jealousy and unhappy – Africa!

Now – What? When Real COVID arrives?!

Whilst Europe still has its populations, with representation in numbers and wellness in all its generations, as visible in congregations and gatherings, the following is the first best thing for us in Africa:

May God talk to African leaders.

May the Creator of the Heavens and Earth influence leadership in Africa more than ever.

May the children of Zimbabwe and Africa give good-heed to the Word of God as God gives us another chance to live to His will.

May the The Lord of the Universe sharpen the minds of scholars and students of Universities of Africa into thinking and planning and work-strategy, doing all things in the reverence of God for real business solutions for Africa and beyond.

May God help African parents to rear and up-bring their seed with seeds of life based on God's order for Africa, be it plant or animal life

May God help doctors of Africa to re-think and re-learn the African way for the survival of Africa!

May the 'lawyers' of Africa revisit the diluted and scraped haven of laws and rules and precepts that preserved the African, and were reinforced by the Holy Word of God in their conservative and preserving ways for sound living in a balanced ecosystem, physically to psychosocially.

May God bequeath upon Africans the love for their own heritage of productive **value.**

May God remind Africa, of His Love for the penitent, and how His Son and Moses once survived therein.

May God remove from this surface, those who do not turn away from creating biological weapons meant to eliminate populations that may turn back to Him, and turn the weapons against them and their non-repenting populations.

May God give Africa another chance for a healthy and orderly reproductive era, for healthy seed unto sound respectful living, free from condom-traps, vaccine-traps, family planning-traps, GMO-food traps, fertilizer and Agrochemical-traps, and other hidden killers from lethal formulae by covetous nations.

79

May God bless Africa with an HIV/AIDS-free generation.

May God stay the enemy's Corona virus plans from destroying African populations.

May God block downloads of evil programs down to Africa.

May God deal in His own ways of Wisdom with Africans who mediate and enable the killing strategies of the enemy over Africa, whether the fellow African 'agents' are doing it out of ignorance or deliberately whilst knowing, due to money cover-ups and terrible bribes.

May He bless and preserve our young ones and lads/lasses and the rest of youth.

May He bless our remaining few elderly to mind their last days for the sake of the younger ones.

May God indeed show Africa, His way of Salvation.

May God prove to Africa the **freedom** from His Salvation.

Amen

The end to my story.

Next – testimonials and plates and other illustrations.

Then the **Epilogue**.

TESTIMONIAL 1

WS

'Here I arrive at our common residence, not the least in my mind that strange news is in wait for me. Entering in at the gate, the hour – early eventide, other residents surround fires in the open yard as they still man their pots over the simple traditional fireplaces.

Immediately, all of them voice out – "*Don't get into the house as yet!*" upon which I question: "Is everything okay?"

"*You are the one who communes and works with Doc; he has the COVID virus, and is in a coma at the Central hospital. When were you two last together?*"

Soon I developed this feeling: **Suddenly Day scares more than Night** – while darkness turns out farer than daylight!

All these people meant I also had the disease. And they insist: "*We don't want to die – let's go to the hospital and get tested!*"

My response: "Well, right now, I'm from a funeral!' And in I entered the house, and straightway into my apartment.

Within a few days, I was to go and trim Gogo's hedge (*Gogo* is traditional reverent-address for Doc's mother). Passersby from the neighborhood would greet me in wonder – as if expressing: "*Why? – Isn't he aware, the residents of this homestead have COVID 19?*"

And their stare signified it all the more vividly: "*Poor fool, so ignorant, even to the point of death!*"

Then I had eventually to visit a friend (who had sent a message through his cellphone) and I had to really examine him: "What is the implication of your message?"

And his response: *"It has been reported – Doc has deceased at the Central hospital – these are the rumors around – and I trust you've got the full story"*

And I told him straight: "Doc is alive!" and he was shocked, for the word had gone round strongly!

At this point I recall a rumored prayer of a German man which is said to have gone this wise (sort of weird, but bearing significance):-

'God, protect me from my friends;
As for my enemy, I will face him on my own!'

TESTIMONIAL 2

GI

'When the testing team arrived, they tested me in the open, by the doorstep! Because of their work-garments, they attracted and drew a crowd from the roads – there was no privacy!

People said: "*That man has COVID!*"

Some shouted: "*He has brought COVID to our township!*"

Soon, a village health worker (*vhw*) addressed a gathering at the Community Borehole saying that, there was someone with 'Corona' within the area….

Following this I heard a lot of passersby *pointing* aloud: "*There is someone with 'Corona' at this house!*"

At one instance, someone from our immediate locality went to a tuckshop – they denied his money: "*It needs to be sanitized first!*" they said, eventually 'waving' him off: "*Sorry! We have no change!*"

When the second tests were due, the COVID team alerted me of their imminent visit; I had to positively suggest, that they have the sample taken at the clinic than at home.

One striking observation, not to be missed: the health workers would stand 5metres away whilst talking to me. I had to enquire: "Why? Wouldn't this stigmatize the people?"

And their excuse: They were not fully equipped with proper work-garments!

My family, even my little children, could so easily notice the breakdown between myself and the community! A new era had dawned – a time that most seemed would never again associate with me, except a few!'

TESTIMONIAL 3

Gogo Gwatidzo (Retired Teacher)

'I was busy watering the front-yard garden, when an ambulance fully-packed with people stopped by the gate. How excited they were, as if they were coming from soccer! The one driving asked:

"Is this Dr Gwatidzo's place?"

I said: "Yes"

Everyone in the ambulance came out excited. By the driver's mentioning – Dr Gwatidzo – I thought: "My son is no more……"

I was trembling.

One asked me: "Did he phone you?"

I said: "No."

He said with 'confidence': "Dr Gwatidzo wabatwa Corona virus" meaning "Dr Gwatidzo has been found to have the Corona virus."

I tell you, I nearly collapsed; but thank God – HE was with me. By that time, all of them were in the yard. They looked very happy and excited. Neighbors also watched and saw from afar. It was my first time to see people from the hospital so excited about a disease!

I thought: "These are the people who should understand how to **counsel**! Talking about COVID 19 right at the gate! This excitement was apparently injected by the conduct of the local hospital's chief-doctor! Lack of professionalism was displayed!

One with a spray-tank/pump sprayed the toilet – how horrible the entire procedure – myself being an asthmatic!

But there were two exceptional ladies on the team – very dignified; they didn't say much, rather than testing me.

How worried I was now? I will not forget this. In anguish, I viewed the doctor who had inflicted a wound in my 'body'! How was this going to heal? Each time we do things, let's engage our brains before opening the mouth. How stressed I am – since that day?! I thought medical practitioners are the ones who **counsel** people or patients – they are viewed as the cream of the nation – isn't it so?

Everyday a pair would then come to visit us. But nothing like COVID was found, in test or in disease form. After publishing all this to the whole world! What is this local hospital doctor going to do about all this? Publishing abroad something that has no certainty! I wanted to talk to him, but he never came.

I remember the Scripture: **The fear of the Lord is the beginning of wisdom**

At our Garden Centre, this chief-doctor and his company, were met at the gate by Dr Gwatidzo's son. This is what the chief-doctor said to Dr Gwatidzo's son:

"Mudhara wako arohwa neCovid 19.….Unoiziva Covid 19?"

And the minor (an eleven year old) answered:

"All I know is – my father was suffering from Malaria."

'Playing' with something that is very serious is not good.

Here is the rule: Tell no lies! But expose lies whenever they are told. Nothing is more satisfying than doing 'good' to others.

Since that day, I'm not myself. I'm always in prayer, so that I can overcome – people now 'fear' us. You see how terrible it is. Think about that – if it was you! If you would like to read Mark 7v20to23.'

TESTIMONIAL 4(INTERVIEW FORMAT)

GM

D: *"What do those people say today Gogo, who said you should not fetch water from the borehole?"*

GM: "It's all over now! A-a-ah! It's all over now! After all, what can they say now, seeing we are living and walking?"

"I simply told them, well, I have no disease, I was tested, and my entire family was tested too – actually you might be the ones with that disease, since you are all not tested; as for myself I'm proven to be okay."

D: *"Really, you gave them a well-thought and wonderful response!"*

GM: "Yes, I told them, we have all been tested, and all of them at work have been tested, and no one has been found to have the disease!"

D: *"But tell me Gogo – who exactly had barred you from getting water from the borehole?"*

GM: "My grandchildren reported, that they were inhibited with strong word, as they tried to get water from the borehole being told: 'Go away, otherwise you contaminate and spread to us the COVID which your granny brought from her workplace!'"

D: *"Who said these words to them Gogo, other children or some elderly people?"*

GM: "A-a-ah, some Elderly people!

"One of these days I met them whilst returning from work, and they asked: 'How then, Gogo *va* Kenny, we no longer see you these days?' to which I responded: 'Where can you see me, for I'm at home or at work?!'"

"And they continued: 'We realize you no longer visit us?!' upon which I answered them: 'Isn't it you said I have COVID, and isn't it you stopped my grandchildren from drawing water from the borehole? So I have been rising up in the twilight, draw my water, and stay in my yard!'"

"Then they started refuting, upon which I suggested to them that, anyway, it was 'probably their children' who barred my grandchildren, then I left it at that!"

D: "*How about the Village Headman? Did he say anything?*"

GM: "A-a-ah, No, he didn't ask even a 'little'. In fact no one would dare to come to our homestead then! All would just eschew or pass by without greeting us."

D: "*But today, have you asked them why they are now coming again? And are there any who have come even to ask for salt?*"

GM: "I never ask them, kkkkk, why would I? As for salt, they began to come much later!"

"These people, got to the extent of spreading news that I had been carried by ambulance to the Central hospital! So one of these mornings, I see my cousin-brother, come on a bicycle, having been sent by one of our fathers to see who was now minding the children. And he was surprised to find me at home. I told him – I hadn't gone anywhere – and that an ambulance indeed did come – we were just tested – and I remained home with the children."

"Another sister in law, who has trouble with legs, phoned and wanted to come – I had to stop her, till I accosted her and explained the position!"

D: "*Let me tell you something Gogo: Inno's neighbor's money was refused at the tuckshop?!*"

GM: "As for myself, I only went to the shops before the 'day'! And the shop-attendant said: 'Ah! Gogo, your doctor is ill, we have heard', and it troubled me and I asked how she had known. I tried to dodge her enquiry, but she knew even much, even the fact that the doctor was admitted at the Central Hospital, and that 'yesterday he tested positive to COVID'! I told her that all I knew was that our doctor had been admitted with Malaria. I enquired as to her source of information, and she responded that the local hospital chief-doctor had sent her a phone message with that information. She said that upon hearing that message, she awoke her husband, shared with him with concern about Gogo's grandchildren, and the fact that Gogo too could have contracted COVID herself. She granted immediately that her heart beat fast upon seeing me."

"And I insisted, really, that's what the hospital chief-doctor told you? He really sent you a message? And she conceded."

"The following day another fellow showed me some pictures, whereby there was a coffin, supposed to bear the body of Dr Gwatidzo, with people surrounding"

D: "*Ha-ha-ha-ha-ha-ha-a-a-a!*"

GM: "She did eventually took my money, I trust only because we are related – but others who would come, they would have to wash their hands thoroughly before she served them; she refused to answer phone calls on the handsets of buyers whose husbands wanted to negotiate about grocery and intending to pay with electronic money – insisting they should call on her own phone directly!"

"And I told her, all I knew: our doctor had been admitted with Malaria – upon which she insisted, I would see hospital cadres coming to test us in our homestead on the day; and surely they came!"

"I didn't know how to explain to children to prepare them, who soon alerted me of an ambulance calling in the yard; and was surprised – so they tested us eventually, all of us, and they did some spraying as per the word of the shop-lady!"

D: "*So that lady knew, even to be sure that they would come on the day, to do some tests and even to spray? How is she related to the chief hospital doctor – are they friends?*"

GM: "She really knew! But as for their relationship, I wouldn't know"

D: "*Did the doctor come?*"

GM: "No he didn't come, and this particular team was not to return; follow up to the end was done by another pair that came daily till they 'finished'"

D: "*But Gogo tell me, if true COVID disease arrives with its effects, will these hospital cadres continue to run around with this kind of work they are doing?*"

GM: "Never!"

D: "*By the way Gogo you went to one of your fathers' funeral recently, did you get to the burial?*"

GM: "In the end, my brothers called me and told me that they had phoned and spoken to my doctor, and heard he was fine – we reconciled well and they dismissed the attitudes of people and the chief doctor, whom they said had sent hateful messages to the people within their own community too!"

D: *"Indeed your brothers did phone me Gogo! But why would this chief-doctor do that Gogo, even to mention the name of the doctor who tested positive?"*

GM: "I don't understand either!

EPILOGUE

COVID 19 has stemmed from hatred to effect hate. The first chapter of Proverbs, the eleventh to the fourteenth verses, bear the intentions to be effected by the WICKED who have planned COVID and whosoever shall be their recruits in sharing their wicked activities:

11. "....**Come with us, let us lay wait for blood, let us lurk privily for the innocent without cause:**
12. **Let us swallow them up alive as the grave: and whole, as those that go down into the pit:**
13. **We shall find all precious substance, we shall fill our houses with spoil:**
14. **Cast in thy lot among us; let us all have one purse**

And sounds like a 'New World Order' committee for the WNE planning to form a new government to loot Africa in the absence of black people's voices! Will The God of The Heavens permit this?

Anyway, I'm not so much to dwell on that in this epilogue. But before I go on to the target of this epilogue, I shall show you the advice of a wise parent to her son/daughter, again from the same scripture – Proverbs 1v10&15 below. And so, who is wise? Who shall be obedient?

Verse 10: **My son, if sinners entice thee, consent not.**

Verse 15: **My son, walk not thou in the way with them: refrain thy foot from their path:**

And before I close this 'little bit', wouldn't Africa be the BIRD here to escape:

Verse 17: **Surely in vain the net is spread in the sight of any bird.**

And given the value to God of the 'smallest bird', why not repent Africa like Nineveh and earn love and protection from the Creator of the Universe:

Matthew 10v 29to31

> **29. Are not two sparrows sold for a farthing? And one of them shall not fall on the ground without your Father.**
> **30. But the very hairs of your head are all numbered.**
> **31. Fear ye not therefore, ye are of more value than many sparrows.**

If only Africans would renounce all evils from 'exports' and from within – and uphold God's Gospel of repentance – the result is God's protection in His Salvation.

Let us now go to the main aim of this Epilogue – for we ought not to leave the seeker at a loss – one should be at least equipped on how to prepare for this era of COVID – no effort is too late!

COVID THREAT? – **HELP!**

I. Promotion of health

1. <u>Constitutional living</u> – our NFH Wellness Restoration manual, has tried to address this issue in a nutshell. Even snakes know their constitution and you will not need to teach them what to eat and what not to eat. Humans have been cheated, spoiled, abused and corrupted! Correction means no sugar and no hormones etc. Hence most commercial provisions, will be out of the question, including milks & meats & ova sold as 'eggs' & 'drinks'. Otherwise load yourself with Vitamin C containing local fruits which run a lengthy 'season' even throughout winter, including **Masawu** (Ziziphus mauritania), plus some well-adapted introduced fruit like Guava! Half a lemon squeezed into every glass of drinking water is a good daily regular. Baobab fruit added to traditional cereal juice, even *Mahewu*, is excellent.

2. <u>Fix the bone+</u> - This is the chief industrial site for the manufacturing of blood with its full white-cell components for defense – marrow being full of fat, it must be provided with constitutional oils from **goat meat** and complete small grains especially **Bulrush millet** (mhunga) – roasted but not put through a de-hurler. Given additions from local forest fruits, the entire defense (including the inert and lymphatics) is fixed. The 'firing' glands for energy mobilization + use (endocrine) & the digestive glands (paracrine) are both fixed.

3. Cleanse the liver/pancreatic system – local herbal teas including the bitter ones correct this bile-reliant system – for maintenance of proper liver & pancreatic function. Bile is an effective sterilizer and where the stomach lacks enough acid, worse still if the liver-gall bladder-pancreatic system is inadequate, the combination is a disaster – predisposing to infections and breakdown of defense. With increased infections and infestations, the gut/intestinal 'lymphatics' are challenged beyond their protective function. Drink lemon juice and bitter teas. NFH have a special bitter tea. An example of a common bitter plant of similar effect, but consumed in a different way is naturally grown lettuce, even as a salad. The spleen in turn is cleansed and toned too.

4. Strengthen and enhance the reins for cleansing –most people in this era have their kidneys compromised, with a high rate complicating to warrant dialysis. The best drink in the world is water – but it should be sound clean water not packaged chemical-laden water or 'sewer water'. At NFH they have an overall natural 'cleanser' and restorer with the trade code – **TSN**. At a low dose, a monthly course will help the kidneys to be toned and charged for their cleansing function; but this should be combined with sound adherence to wellness-living principles.

II. Prevention of disease

1. Household herbs – oral: Onion boiled every evening for 5 minutes in 500mls of water is good for the Upper & Lower Respiratory tracts. The onion water cooled, may be dropped into both ears

too. Corn/Maize silk as from a single maize cob can be boiled in 500mls and taken once daily for not more than 7days, for cleansing the kidneys (of infections) and the entire urinary tract. For the **R**espiratory Tract and the **R**eins (R & R) have to be especially toned against challenges of Corona viruses!

2. Household herbs – inhalational: This form of practice may be preventive plus additional to corrective therapy. **Leaves** of Zumbani (Lippia Javanica), Lemon, Guava and Eucalyptus, may be boiled together to saturation – the vapor is inhaled as in a fomentation from a cup on a table or a bigger vessel (without covering the head please – not necessary here!). This may be done for 5 days once or twice daily, skipping a week in between, each session lasting for the period till the vapour is finished. Caution: It should be ensured that the Eucalyptus is from a naturally grown plantation!

3. Productive Exercise: Grow your own culinary and useful herbs and vegetables in lovely beds + Haitian-bags and pots, finding soil and watering them with small size cans, whilst walking fast or non-strenuous running – and not walk around the dangerous roads without extra-benefit. Avoid garden workers, or if you have one, never allow them to do your own portion for you. He may gather rocks and soils and composts from outside for you; but pack your own polybags and vases etc., sow and manage them on a working-daily basis. Train your children similarly. For office workers & school-goers, 15 – 30 minutes of such productive exertion, yields great and almost adequate exercise for the body per day. Exercise tones the body's defense, let alone exercise which produces nutrients in the garden.

4. Office Workers & Sunshine: This class of workers suffer incomplete Vitamin D metabolism, which is especially vital for defense against viral respiratory challenges etc. They spent most of their day in the shade. At break and lunch time, they should have their natural snack or victual whilst strolling in the sun; terrible hot commercial tea and coffee whilst in the same office-shade is a disaster over long periods of time! With the sun, the bone is complete for providing defense components too. Black-skinned people in the temperate

climates may have a worse challenge for sure due to this Vitamin D fact.

III. Treatment of Early Stages

1. Leaves ZLGEA oral – a handful each of leaves of, **Z**umbani, **L**emon, **G**uava, **E**ucalyptus and **A**vocado – boiled in a litre of water for 15minutes, is a useful adopted formula in the treatment of Corona viruses in our Southern African region. Ask people of Malawi and Zimbabwe, they will tell you the same, especially for the first four. The Avocado leaf will aid further with the red-blood-cell nutrient-component of iron for the hemoglobin complex. Remember the Oxygen carrying-capacity of blood is vital in Respiratory affections.

2. Counter coagulation – Garlic + Artemisia: The **garlic** bulb is made up of segments called cloves. 3 cloves of organic garlic are blended into 250mls of water (stronger concentration), or cut and naturally infused into 125mls of water over 12 hours (where a blender is not available). The 125mls is drunk every morning and every evening, within an hour after a good meal. Caution: Do not swallow garlic cloves – and alley the risk of possible gastric irritation or even ulceration. Each region bears characteristic plants, at times represented in each continent. Africa has its own **Artemisia *afra*,** very safe for humanity and a sound treatment against Malaria for all prone age-groups. China has its own Artemisia *annua*, again studied over years and with preparations well-formulated or established for Malaria treatment. But there is great value hidden too in the useful teas of these plants for COVID 19 – their capacity to prevent clot formation without risk of causing bleeding in the body. It is important to be traditionally or professionally guided in dosages in drinking the teas. One has to be careful with other varieties of Artemisia, especially A. *absinthium*, with regard to extremes of age and vulnerability of certain adult patients of a weaker disposition, e.g. to stomach-ulceration.

3. Renal reinforcement – AFUDLC + MSP: This special empirically based formulation and combination by NFH, well known for

healing severe forms of **H1N1** in the experiences of our practice over the past 13years, achieves amazing healing capacity in its ability to restore the breathing apparatus and tone the kidneys. Recovery of the afflicted may dawn within 24 hours! It is the principle that is important!

4. Warmth (x7) & hot rich liquid-foods: It is essential to keep these patients very warm. It wouldn't be a surprise to lose a patient from severe Hypothermia in cases of heavy Corona-virus infestations. Where a hearth is available, the patient should be moved to such a new 'bedroom', and the fire kept burning especially overnight. Safe hot-water bottles are essentially needful with an attendant to ensure their warmth imparting capacity is consistently maintained.

IV.   Prescription class and complications

1. AFUDLC + MSP: This author has an example even with his own mother, sometime in September 2019, when she suffered a severe form of Influenza Type A pattern of illness, indeed H1N1 in pattern – we nearly lost her. It was this AFUDLC & MSP combination from NFH that saved her. The attack and deterioration had been fast. She had come off a wedding gathering, where she had not lasted more than 15minutes as she was only to give a special present to her former student. Within 24hours, she complained of heavy dyspnea, so unusual with related body weakness. She mentioned this was beyond her former Asthma attacks. A cough was present and progressive, but no coryza. Headaches and fever reigned, with severe chills. She suddenly ran into complications while we thought it was a passing 'flu', hardly capable due to breathlessness to manage up to toilet! The hearth and the NFH formulation was to save her at the point many were concerned she might not last that Friday night, whereby the Devil was trying to persuade me to believe that I was waiting for her last breath. Midnight, she surprisingly rose up to the bathroom, emptied her bowels, returned and exclaimed: 'Really? Is that I, to walk myself like this?!' And Saturday's sun smiled at her basking outside in fresh air from the trees in the yard. I have often told:

'Had she gone to a ventilator – it would have been another story'! Then, I had not the least idea of the COVID 19 reports around the Eastern corner, 3+ months away!

2. Get to a well-ventilated area: The living room where we transferred our mother's bedroom to is an expanse full of fresh air; and had it not been the hearth consistently loaded with aptly cut pieces of well-dried firewood (prepared by my loving son Frank), the room would have been deadly cold. I was the only one with her up to her wonderful recovery about midnight, as I kept an even fire. When she struggled with a seeming last 'rough' & 'tough' breath, and became **silent**, I thought that was her last, as I kept my bolding head down! A minute later, when I raised my brows, I watched her in amazement as she evenly breathed restfully and unobstructed, to sleep calmly for about two hours - this was the point she awoke – and I wouldn't believe myself when she got herself down the bed in good balance, and with ease, and steadily walked down the corridor, and right into the toilet at the far end. And she returned and exclaimed the restoration of her wellness that has lasted to this day, even to see and suffer with her son, this most recent 'false COVID' ordeal that the Lord permitted me to go through while I was burdened with Resistant Malaria!

3. Keep very warm: I indeed I and my son and loved ones kept Mum warm. My sister's visit from the UK had fortuitously left us with a gift of a special resilient hot-water bottle and its 'safety-jacket' to prevent scalds. Together with fire and a warm bed, plus the hearth in the last days, The Lord saw her through! Drinking water, healing teas & medicines plus foods, are best given very warm to hot.

4. Massaging, hot dry-baths & 'physio': During Mum's illness, our 'home-hospital' was grossly short of staff – only my son and I! My 11+year old son had to grow in mind and physique and stature as in a moment, while God capacitated him in love and longsuffering and loving-kindness to serve his grandmother – Gogo! This quality was to be evident too at the time of my illness. Being 'men', both of us, we wouldn't help Mum to the best with physio, but we did our minimum. This is so essential, to aid the circulation into all

tissues, organs and organ-systems without impediment. Pressure sores get out of the question when mobilization, passive and active is started early and maintained. For dry baths, the towel has to be dipped into very hot water and wrung to express all drops. Adding aloe to the water (+/- some salt crystals) is grossly beneficial.

MALARIA! MALARIA! MALARIA!

How can I close this story without 'folding up' the last page with a note on Malaria!

The recent attack was the second in my life (at age 52years) – the first having been when I was 14/15years of age. I must tell my dear Reader: THE PATTERN OF MALARIA HAS CHANGED IN AFRICA!

And I don't believe that it's all from the story of 'resistance' that we are told. For now the world being fraught of fraudster-virologists, why would it lack rotten 'falciparumologists' and 'Anopheletologists' who can corrupt the ecosystems with lab-generated strains for evil intention upon humans created by God, yet they deem them unnecessary on the earth's surface unto a covetous end! One would doubt to doubt the Burkina Faso story about mosquitoes!

I did not delay in having my illness with Malaria treated. But I followed the treatment protocol on our own natural line, which has saved my patients without limitations. Yet this time around, I had not realized that, strains of P. falciparum along the Mozambican belt are even up to a stubborn menace now. It was never like that with my travelers. I speculate on what predisposed me, being a non-sugar eater, but even on the oranges I blame, I'm not yet fully-convinced they are the culprits. I fear there's another lurking factor. For on correct diet alone, whilst traversing borders, I have never contracted Malaria. 52years – 14years = 38years free of Malaria attacks! What suddenly makes me prone to Malaria?

Now the surrounding areas of Zimbabwe are not 'quiet'! Immediate areas in the vicinity and distally within our district of Murewa suffer a 'soring' epidemic to this day, with possibly an undoubted record death-rate! Distant areas, including Mutoko and Mudzi (the area adjacent to Mozambique border, where I picked my strain) are all registering unknown rates and 'rages' of lethal Malaria.

Yet, when it comes to the death-causality, one has to be very careful: Treatment with the Coartem tablets availed in our public systems, has often resulted in severe hypoglycaemic attacks which can consume the patient's life earlier than the Malaria itself. Before my attack with Malaria, our beloved New, Newton, had one serious one which nearly took his life. He suffered 3 hypoglycaemic attacks we struggled with in the garden; and even in my presence as a doctor, I witnessed them to be formidable. I imagined an old lady staying with grandchildren, in our 'orphan-land', and wondered how she would cope in a hypoglycaemic attack of a Malaria-sufferer on Coartem, when she can't even diagnose it, let alone have ever heard about it or known it! It simply means loss of life! From Malaria? No! From Coartem!

Our African governments and Medical and Wellness ministries have to be alerted here! We need to promote research on and production of simple empirical formulae of teas from natural plants that alleviate the hazard of Malaria in the way of extensive Agricultural and Therapeutic programs, that promote and avail adequate solutions even to be exported, rather than import and use alien preparations, whilst sitting in offices and treatment-centres without realizing the risk on our populations of 'foreign materials'!

COVID TESTING AND MALARIA!

My case alone of a Positive Malaria Test, and a '*Positive*' PCR COVID test, makes my mind warrant a study for this COVID 19 *type* of testing on all cases of Malaria – for I feel there's such a high possibility of false positives, and mind you, not from Malaria alone, but many other conditions.

Such studies should be set-aside for devoted scholars – money mongers are too busy for such – and their brains are saturated with covetousness. Some of them hazarded (if they had not decided deliberately) killing me by stopping my Malaria treatment for two days, whilst enclosing me in a hospital ward, never nearby to communicate a word to me!

But it is important to note that a combination of the real COVID 19 disease (when its importation gets truly effected) and the current raging MALARIA, given their almost similar mode of complication, the resultant disease-complex would be unbearably devastating!

And I remind you:

WHEN COVID REALLY ARRIVES, YOU SHALL KNOW BY THE HEARSES ON THE ROAD, AND BY RISING SMOKES SIGNIFYING DEATHS IN THE VILLAGES AND IN TOWNS!

Then the money mongers and scoffers and scorners and arrogant will be silenced.

Let us pray: As happened with EBOLA to this day – God stays COVID19 **Disease** from arriving into Southern Africa!

Positive-test is not necessarily equal to disease, especially at this point in time!

Yet stay alert and be careful.

Good Bye!

INTERESTING AFTER-REMARKS

Kuswe Covid remarks off a mask-less officer

17-6-2020 1320hrs

Arrival at Kuswe clinic - 1st port = COVID desk

A short but bulk of a figure pushing a stomach in white long sleeved 'Covid' shirt plus black trousers makes amazing recognition....

And his remarks above a naked beard, no mask:

'Ndivo vapfanha vakandiitisa mari ava' translating **'These are the young men that earned me sums of money without sweat'** as he approaches the bench and the patient without the slightest social distancing rule!

Oh, that money-motive! He looked to us like a COVID extension officer on the Environmental Health Technician roll. And he even salutes our *'Nomore'* by name! Bit-coin memory?!

I'm glad we haven't introduced ourselves - myself and Frank having remained behind and stuck to the 'car-chassis'.

Even more interesting, he dissuades his assistant from performing a COVID test. Very smart for both parties! Why? Otherwise another false-positive would have re-pushed all of us all-over-again into the Corrupt-COVID-pool!

He had ranted and chanted: "high fever + headache = most probable **Malaria....!"**

o   And the man demonstrated recognition beyond just familiarity of a subject he had followed-up on my positive test!

o   So how would it taste if another truly positive Malaria-test would influence another impact of a false-positive COVID test?!

As we reverse and pull-off, I'm glad to hear Nomore's response that the man hasn't made inquiry of us, for introduction of ourselves never have we done! I guess they just considered us as 'hire-offerers' of a 'Matatu'!

9 781665 506106